Your Personal Health Guide

The Secret To Gaining *And Maintaining* Health

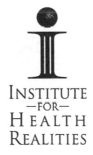

INSTITUTE
—FOR—
HEALTH
REALITIES

Institute for Health Realities, 5245 Centennial Blvd., Suite 100, Colorado Springs, CO 80919, web site: http://www.healthrealities.org
(formerly Queen and Company health communications, inc.)

Made in the United States of America.

TO THE READER

CAUTION: The writings contained in this book are meant as a source of information, and are not intended to provide individual medical advice. Such advice must be obtained from a qualified practitioner.

International Standard Book Number (ISBN): 0-9620479-4-5

Who is Sam Queen?

H.L. "Sam" Queen, M.A., C.C.N., D.Sc.(hon.) President and founder of the Institute for Health Realities, is a Certified Clinical Nutritionist. He has had over 30 years in the health care field; first as a medical technologist where he learned how to understand and interpret blood results; then as an author and investigative medical reporter, where he learned how to access the most up-to-date medical research available in the field of diet and lifestyle; then as a health care educator, which enabled him to put all of it together and teach health professionals what he knew. Finally, as a Certified Clinical Nutritionist he has developed a unique talent for connecting blood chemistries with diet and lifestyle, drawing upon the total of this information to improve the health and lives of many. As the developer of *Free Radical Therapy* and the *BioDesign Model of Health™*, Mr. Queen–along with his entire staff–is ready to assist you in your quest for improved health!

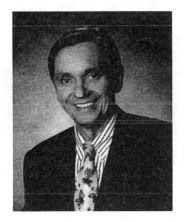

Table of Contents

Introduction
The Purpose Of This Guide

If you want to improve your health, you face a confusing maze of options. This booklet is intended to guide you through that maze by addressing the realities that are required for your health.

Perhaps the most important reality, and the one you must consider first is that *we believe the body was made by design, not by accident.* Health is possible only by gaining a thorough understanding of your body's design and then developing a strategy to support that design.

The alternative is to believe otherwise: That your body was made by accident, and that disease and poor health are due to an unfortunate gene pool from which resulted a series of flaws. Looking at your health from this mind-set is how medicine is generally practiced today. As a result, the strategies of today's standard of care are aimed at dictating to your body through drugs and surgery rather than supporting its natural design. This helps explains your difficulty in getting well using the contemporary health care system, and why this personal health guide is so important.

Another important reality is that health goals cannot be achieved without first defining the target. You might know generally where you want to go with your health (freedom from disease, pain, and low energy), but if you don't know how to get there–and if your health provider is no better prepared–then it's probable you won't reach your destination. As simple as this seems, it is generally not applied. Instead, today's health care system tends to veer away from true health because the system and its proponents have a very shortsighted view of what comprises health.

Considering this, the results are not surprising. If you adopt the assumption that the body is made by accident, then health is a myth, not a reality. At best, it is looked upon only as the absence of disease and risk factors. Such a definition is limp, and by its nature leads to weak results.

We are on a mission to better define your health target, remove myth, and aid you in your pursuit of optimum health.

The process of defining your health target leads us to persistently and passionately seek answers to the question, "What constitutes health?"

The definition of health, the road that leads there, and how to get there from *your* present position, requires (as you might expect) multifaceted answers. Rather than keeping our findings a secret until all the answers are determined, we have developed all kinds of ways to help you benefit *now*. Some of our methods include the *Health Realities Journal*™, textbooks, audiocassettes, videotapes, and seminars where we train your doctor to apply the required concepts.

In order to test the practical nature of our findings, and at the same time allow you to actually use this information, we also provide health consultations. Of necessity, these consultations are restricted to those who join our HealthConnection Action Group, becoming familiar with the required concepts and thereby facilitating our quest.

In summary, then, *Your Personal Health Guide* serves three primary purposes:

1. It provides you with credible, straightforward answers to solving disease and infections. Once you've read this booklet, you'll be better equipped to work with the Institute for Health Realities or a Free Radical Therapy practitioner. By gaining a better understand-

ing of our philosophy beforehand, it stands to reason that you can expect a better outcome.

2. It shows you how to get ongoing support to satisfy your continuing health needs.

3. It's a directory of all of the health resources, services, and products available from the *Institute for Health Realities*. You'll find answers to why these products and services have been chosen, how they interrelate, and how they can be of help to you in your own personal quest for health.

Chapter One
What We Can Do For You

At the Institute for Health Realities, we've helped people gain: more energy, vitality and a greater sense of well-being; stronger resistance to disease; and solutions for existing health problems...in short, better health!

We can help you overcome the effects of accumulated hazardous materials exposure, which in itself may be an important cause of poor health. Or, if you and your health care practitioner have already undertaken a treatment plan which hasn't generated the desired results, we can help you improve those results.

In addition, we can help you and your health care practitioner address the underlying accumulation of toxic agents which may be interfering with your current treatment plan.

If you're not suffering from contaminant materials exposure, we can still help you raise your current level of health well beyond what you might attain by addressing "risk factors" only. We do this by tailoring your diet and lifestyle to fit your personal needs, which includes consideration of your blood chemistry pattern.

Am I Exposed To Hazardous Materials?

You may be surprised to discover that most people have toxic substance exposures built into their lives.

These exposures come from a great many sources. One that has received a significant amount of media coverage is mercury from dental amalgam fillings. Most adults and many children in America have amalgam restorations.

Mercury from amalgam isn't the only exposure for most people, however, and it is certainly not the only commonly encountered hazardous material.

Since the industrial revolution began just 300 years ago mankind has introduced into the environment over 100,000 new metal and chemical combinations that had never before existed. (This was reported in the series "A Prescription for Health" published in our quarterly *Health Realities Journal*.) Many of these substances are regarded as contaminant or hazardous materials–the volume often exceeding your body's ability to neutralize them. This is important to each and every one of us, because no one is immune to toxic exposures. The result is that virtually everyone has now been contaminated to some degree or another.

The source of these unhealthy contaminant exposures can generally be categorized into the following four major groups:

1. Heavy metals such as lead, copper, tin, cadmium and mercury.
2. Pesticides such as dieldrin and DDT.
3. Organic solvents like cleaning fluids, varnish stripping agents, and formaldehyde.
4. Drugs, petrochemicals, and other man-made agents like antibiotics and gasoline, along with the by-products of these agents, such as carbon monoxide.

Collectively and individually, these agents are a part of each of us, and serve as strong catalysts of free radical formation–by-products of oxidation that cause premature deterioration of the human body and its many parts. They turn perfectly healthy cholesterol into something labeled "bad," promote aging, lower your resistance to infection, and bring about (or make worse) nearly all chronic disease situations.

Free radical exposure occurs in other ways, as a common result of our way of life. Deep-fried foods are suspect. Some fast food restaurants change the cooking oil in their deep fat fryers infrequently. This can become a "breeding ground" for free radical exposure.

What Are Free Radicals?

Free radicals result from the process known as oxidation. In oxidation, energy is produced at the expense of altering the oxidizing agent or oxidative substrate in such a way as to leave either or both with an unpaired (and highly energized) electron in the outer electron orbit. The problem is that these highly energized, unpaired electrons are like microscopic tornadoes. They roam through their cellular neighborhoods looking for a matching electron to steal at the expense of ripping apart whatever gets in the way.

In your healthy body, antioxidants come to the rescue to try and intercept the tornado before it can do harm. However, when the number of toxic materials (acting as oxidant catalysts) outnumber the antioxidant defenses, then free radicals win out, causing what is known as oxidative stress. Subsequently, as the body burden of free radicals grow, the tornadoes grow in number and strength. The cascade of free radicals that follows makes the body particularly susceptible to damage from metals such as mercury, lead, cadmium, copper and iron.

Why Are We Concerned About Free Radicals?

Oxidative stress created by an excess of free radicals relative to the antioxidant defenses–such as may occur when the body burden of chemicals and heavy metals reaches a saturation point–will inevitably cause cell damage. Damage to DNA is among the most serious of alterations, causing mutagenesis and carcinogenesis. This means that free radicals increase the likelihood of cancer and cellular breakdowns, which may then lead to any one of the many chronic diseases.

Free radicals also interfere with protein metabolism, and–by oxidizing the fatty acids located within cell membranes–may substantially alter the permeability of cell membranes. Once this is accomplished, the damage extends to mitochondrial furnaces, leading to extreme loss of energy, impaired cell function, calcification, and (ultimately) cell death.

Through these and other means, free radicals promote aging and contribute to virtually all degenerative, or chronic disease conditions.

An Overwhelming List Of Symptoms And Diseases

Symptoms and diseases associated with various forms of hazardous exposure include:

* allergic reactions (including rashes and other skin irritations)
* arteriosclerosis
* arthritis
* attention deficit disorders (ADD)
* cancer (of various kinds)
* *Candida albicans*
* chronic aches and pains (including headaches and migraines)
* digestive dysfunction
* fibromyalgia
* frequent cold or flu-like symptoms
* heart disease
* kidney and liver diseases
* lack of energy
* low back pain
* lupus (LE)
* memory disorders
* multiple sclerosis (MS)
* osteoporosis
* peculiar taste sensations (including metallic tastes)

- periodontal disease
- respiratory difficulties
- sleep disorders
- unhealthy blood pressure (high or low)
- unhealthy cholesterol levels (high or low)

...to name a few. Thus, through production of free radicals, nearly all disease can be triggered or mimicked by hazardous materials exposures in their numerous forms.

The increased frequency of these symptoms demonstrates that—more than ever before—our environment is a contamination hotbed. It is no longer a question of "will you be exposed?" to hazardous materials. The pressing issue of the day is instead, "Are you prepared to properly deal with these exposures?" Helping you deal successfully with these inevitable exposures is one of our primary goals. How do you detoxify?

It Takes More Than Eliminating Exposure

Eliminating the offending material is generally thought to be an important first step to recovery. This philosophy works quite well for most contaminant sources except exposure to mercury from amalgam fillings (which we'll soon explain further).

Exposure elimination is not the whole picture, however. For starters, eliminating exposure to harmful materials (such as mercury from dental fillings) does not remove the accumulated body burden of these materials. Nor does the removal of the offending substance prepare your body for internal chemistry adjustments which may follow.

As a result, many who have sought to remove toxic materials from their lifestyles have not improved as expected, or—in some cases—have ended up with worse health than when they started.

You might consider the following common experience:

If you put an empty bucket under a running faucet, that bucket–as expected–begins to fill. Turning the faucet off will keep the bucket from filling any further, but will not empty the water that has already accumulated. Emptying the bucket of its contents is, obviously, a separate step which must be undertaken if you want to get rid of the accumulated water.

In much the same way, recovering health from contaminant materials exposure requires emptying the bucket along with turning off the faucet. Often, the latter means that we have to first construct a health "handle" so that the bucket *can* be emptied. As a first step, then, your body must be supported in such a way that it can begin the emptying process. In addition, repairs must be made, and because repair needs differ from person to person, the repair process must be tailored to fit you. Accordingly, recovery requires that the source of the exposure, the accumulated contamination, and your needs all be addressed.

Failure to correctly deal with both exposure and accumulated body burden, is the barrier that appears to block much health progress today. This failure may explain why so many who have symptoms connected with heavy metal exposure do not see more marked improvement subsequent to removal of the offending materials. It also helps explain why, when serious health problems exist, you wouldn't want to seek the help of a doctor whose approach is to simply treat you generically (as just another "average person"). It should be apparent that much more is required.

The Solution

Our solution is based on a health model philosophy that we have named *Free Radical Therapy*. Free Radical Therapy focuses on six fundamental, subclinical defects that we've determined to be present during any chronic disease or chronic infection, and which occur months, sometimes years, before disease becomes evident. These six fundamental defects are:

1. acid stress
2. anaerobic tendency
3. free calcium excess
4. chronic inflammation
5. connective tissue breakdown
6. oxidative stress

By identifying these defects and developing a strategy to correct them based on individual need, a world of health opportunities surfaces that otherwise would not exist.

The Health Model vs. The Disease Model

Decades of research led to the development of the *Health Model* upon which Free Radical Therapy is based. This model is markedly different from the *Disease Model*, which is currently the basis of traditional health practice.

The Disease Model is based on the assumption that health is simply the absence of disease and established risk factors. When medicine is practiced this way, your doctor is expected to assume that disease is mostly the result of flaws in our genetic pool. As a result, the focus of treatment is on making a diagnosis, putting a label on the diagnosis, and then treating the label. This approach works well in crises situations, such as when you've had a heart attack, but it fails miserably when used to handle chronic disease and infections. The flaw rests in the fact that symptoms and risk factors are less often the cause–and more often a reflection–of underlying defects. As a result, treating the symptom by dictating to the body what you would like to have happen– rather than supporting natural mechanisms–does little more than hide the underlying defect.

The Health Model begins, then, with the premise that it is necessary to know how something works in order to repair or improve it. It further proposes that health and lifestyle changes must be addressed from the perspective of their impacts on total health, rather than just focusing on how a procedure impacts a specific symptom.

The Health Model addresses health from a broader framework than the conventional approach. Health is seen, of course, as the absence of disease, and (of course) as the absence of any risk factor that results from bodily abuse. Beyond this, however, health is the absence of any of the six fundamental defects previously described.

Using the Health Model as the starting point, and then looking for those things which violate the model, the relationship of the six fundamental defects to chronic disease and infections becomes apparent.

In addition, addressing the six fundamental defects allows getting at the cause rather than just temporarily eliminating the symptoms. Where disease is not yet present, the Health Model allows the avoidance of future health problems. The focus dramatically shifts from symptom management to supporting natural mechanisms. Symptoms are seen merely as clues generated by the dysfunctioning of one or more of the six health model areas. The secret, then, to long-term success in the handling of symptoms–such as high cholesterol–is to address the six fundamental defects in such a way that the response is tailored to the individual.

The Health Model is, therefore, a frame of reference for both understanding and for attaining health. Through it we gain the new insights which direct us to those steps necessary to not only prevent disease, but also to overcome it.

These concepts are all part of Free Radical Therapy as derived from the Health Model. It is truly a revolutionary approach!

Our Mission

We need to stop here for a moment and note our company's focus. The dramatically new approach to health care management generated by the Health Model results from who we are.

We view the *Institute for Health Realities* not so much as a business, but as a mission. Our mission is help people gain the energy and enthusiasm they need to go about their life's purpose.

That's why we are here, why our clients are both doctors and lay people, and why we want *you* to learn about us.

What About Results?

Using the Health Model-based approach, we've seen some remarkable results. (Among them, that infections can–and usually should–be overcome *without* resorting to antibiotics.)

People with chronic fatigue, sleep disorders, memory difficulties, numerous aches and pains, digestive disorders, chronic depression, systemic impairments, coronary diseases, cancer, autoimmune dysfunctions, and a host of other maladies, have made profound improvements. In each case, however, there were no "magic bullets," no "just give me a pill" cures.

Achieving Change Requires Effort

People like you who've had their "fill" of bad health, began asking the same questions we have researched: "What is good health?" and "What do I have to do to get it?"

More to the point, these individuals abandoned the conventional approach of endless streams of visits to their doctor's offices. They discovered that the standard regimen of drugs and return visits left them without the health they thought they would find. Many of these individuals chose to step off the treadmill.

If you've come to this point, and you're wanting off the treadmill, what can we do for you?

It's important to note here that change isn't always easy–that oftentimes the reason for your health problems lies within a lifestyle "mistake" you probably enjoy! We must remind you that we can only help you within the limits of your willingness to respond.

We can provide you with the key to improving your own health, and guide both you and your doctor in its use. After that, it will be up to you to use it!

Chapter Two: Our Mission
Who We Are...
Where We've Come From...
Where We're Going

If you've visited our web site, you already know something about us. There is much more to know!

Who We Are (And Who We Are Not)

The Institute for Health Realities is the formal name of a company engaged in researching the question "What constitutes optimum health?" We were incorporated as *Queen and Company* in 1988, but our founder, H.L. "Sam" Queen, began his search more than 40 years ago.

Since our formal beginning we've worked with hundreds of you and your doctors. Increasingly we have become a consulting, training and mentoring organization for doctors and their patients.

We are not, however, a medical practice and, accordingly, we do not diagnose or treat disease. This is the job of the licensed doctor. As health consultants we work closely with you and your doctor to develop specific courses of action which are designed to bring about your desired health results.

Why We Focus On Health Communications

You might ask, "If this information is so good, why hasn't my doctor told me about it?" Keep in mind that, as with most new concepts, acceptance is a tedious process. Overcoming commonly accepted misconceptions is a huge task. Just getting the right information in print is a start, but there is a lot more to do.

With more than 30,000 research reports published annually in the health sciences, health care practitioners have a daunting task ahead of them. They don't have time to read even a fraction of what's available, so unless someone is reading and distilling it for them, they are forced to abide by what they're told through national health policy dictates. National health policy is only set after many years of observation. Then, since national health policy is based more on addressing an "average" person rather than specific patients, your unique needs for health pretty much get lost in the shuffle. To help overcome this we publish the *Health Realities Journal*. Through this and our other publications we are literally in the business of trying to "stamp out" truth decay.

Other obstacles remain.

Professional organizations such as the American Medical Association (AMA), American Dental Association (ADA), and American Heart Association (AHA) have severe political and commercial pressures brought upon them–both without and within–to maintain the status quo. The information we hear (officially) from them is only the "party line."

As a result–and even though much of the information we use is derived from the national meetings of these most prestigious medical associations along with the underlying medical literature–we find we must reinterpret almost every finding before it can be applied to health (rather than disease). Thus, most health care practitioners are not aware of the research findings upon which the Health Model and the Free Radical Therapy approach are based. Our publishing efforts and seminar presentations are helping to change this.

A Commercially Barraged Public

The Health Model allows us to apply the findings reported by national "health" organizations and government entities in revolutionary ways. This generates previously unseen results and creates much of the enthusiasm which we see among our clients. Unfortunately, the potential that these extraordinary health improvements hold is all too often wasted. It is difficult for people to avoid being cynical when they are bombarded by the advertising hype and commercialism which is aimed at supporting the quick-fix, crises-oriented, disease model doctrine. If you don't like something, take a pill!

It doesn't take much effort to verify that our airwaves and cable sites are indeed filled with commercials made to look like news reports. The hype from these sources promises to make us successful, fulfilled, give us "abs" of steel, grow hair on our balding heads, and solve problems most of us weren't even aware we had–all with very little effort on our part!

Emphatically, we are not like those companies.

We immediately and categorically distance ourselves from all such efforts: We are not an advertising ploy bent on separating you from your money.

We are first and foremost fully committed to answering the questions "what constitutes health," and, "how was the body designed to repair itself, fight infections, and stay healthy?" Our products and services are designed to share these findings, to help you take advantage of our research, and help you improve your health.

The Wallace Research Foundation's Role In Our Research

To acquire all the information needed in our quest, we first attend the major research meetings, such as the American Heart Association's annual Scientific Sessions, and the annual Experimental Biology meeting. These two meetings alone report over 10,000 findings each year. We also peruse the literature and are constantly doing computer searches of the world's best databases of health information. In addition, we consult directly with researchers and specialists in various health fields. Sam Queen has served for many years as personal research consultant to H.B. Wallace, Administrator of the Wallace Research Foundation (WRF). Through Mr. Wallace and the WRF, he plays an influential role in placing about one million dollars in health research grants each year. And, by virtue of getting to know personally most of the researchers who do this work, Mr. Queen has developed a strong consulting network of health experts. Many of these doctors and researchers make appearances at our seminars. In this way the attendees can gain firsthand knowledge of various topics that are pertinent to health. Through this combined effort, the *Institute for Health Realities* and WRF are seeking to improve the quality of health for all humanity.

The bottom line is: We want to positively affect the health results that are missing from conventional medical treatment.

Where We've Come From

Sam Queen began his health search while working as a medical technician. This research took on a very personal nature when he was diagnosed in 1972 with what was then believed to be an incurable, debilitating disease. Numerous physicians evaluated his condition with the same conclusion: He was terminally ill, and nothing could be done.

Remarkably, he recovered completely!

Why? How? Was God's hand in it? He believes so, but the driving desire to learn the mechanisms by which his illness came about started him on a quest for health answers in general, through the formation of the *Insti-*

tute, and (ultimately) to the discovery of the six sub-clinical defects that separate health from disease and disease risk. Clearly, appropriate attention to those subclinical areas not only creates new opportunities for improved health, but also for the reversal of symptoms and disease labels previously thought untreatable!

Here's a simple example:

The Antibiotic Treadmill

Have you ever had a sinus or ear infection?

You probably went to your doctor, who correctly diagnosed the infection and then prescribed a course of antibiotics.

Like most people, you felt better when you first got on the antibiotics. However, that feeling of well-being probably didn't last. Why?

Most people are unaware that their overall health is directly connected to the acid/base balance of saliva, and to the adequate population and functioning of "friendly" bacteria that populate the intestinal linings. These microorganisms are involved in defending us from disease-causing organisms, and in metabolizing the foods we eat into the nutrients we must have. When your body's pH is correct, these organisms thrive, protect you, and keep you healthy. When your pH is acid, these organisms die.

Within 48 hours of beginning antibiotics, the medicine sterilizes the intestines. In other words, all those healthy bacteria are wiped out. Now, it's true that the infection bacteria (which brought you to your doctor) are probably also destroyed. However your ability to achieve nourishment from the foods you eat became seriously compromised, and your natural defense system was lost.

No wonder you felt good at first, but then felt worse.

And with the death of your friendly bacterial population, it's likely that you soon made a repeat trip to the doctor.

We call this the "antibiotic treadmill." It's relatively easy to overcome, although most doctors don't realize it. It's the kind of answer we've been able to put together for you, and the kind of thing we can help you with.

Where We Are Going

New developments are generating increasingly greater opportunities for you to experience profound health improvements.

To further help you in improving your health we're also working on:

- *A Computerized Health Program*
  To better enable greater numbers of people to have access to health interpretations, we're establishing a computerized health model. Blood chemistries and/or health questionnaires will be analyzed by the computer program. At the Institute new information can be added to the health model as it is published–free of the prejudices and biases that accompany advice from the existing health authorities–rather than waiting for a national committee to amend the accepted standard of care (2-6 years after being published, on average).

- *The HealthConnection Action Group*
  You and your health care professional can gain access to the information as it accumulates by joining our HealthConnection Action Group. If you sign up for our electronic magazine, you'll have access to our latest findings as well as the opportunity to participate in a number of specialized Free Radical Therapy health programs.

- *The Free Radical Therapy Textbook*
  Sam Queen will be adding to and updating this text-book for health care professionals. This detailed ex-planation of the six subclinical defects will be an in-valuable reference book.
- *The Basic One Hundred, A Book Of Chemistry Interpretation*
  This key blood and urine indices textbook provides the necessary resources for those who wish to inter-pret chemistry results from both a Health Model and Disease Model perspective. This book answers many questions that dentists, medical doctors, and other health professionals have in identifying disease, health risks, and the six subclinical defects that un-derlie all diseases and infections. In this book you'll learn how to relate laboratory findings to health com-plaints and health risks, and how to develop a treat-ment strategy. It will also prove helpful and infor-mative to the nonmedical, but keenly-interested stu-dent of health–a source book that can provide the insight needed when trying to persuade a doctor to work with you in implementing the necessary health concepts. A softbound version is now available.
- *The Free Radical Therapy/Mouthful Of Evidence Seminars*
  Basic, Intermediate and Advanced Free Radical Therapy Seminars are scheduled for dentists as well as M.D.'s, D.O.'s and other health professionals. From across the country and around the world, in-creasing numbers of doctors and their team mem-bers are taking these courses and successfully imple-menting the concepts into their practices.

Those interested in finding out more about these products and services are invited to call our office at (719) 598-4968, or log onto our web site at *http:// www.healthrealities.com.*

We're tremendously excited about all of these developments, and would love to share with you all of the information we have gained. Chapter Three will introduce you to some of our existing publications.

Chapter Three:
So You Thought You Were Done With School!

From product labels to books, we encourage you to read and learn. We recommend starting with the labels on the foods and supplements you consume. From there, we encourage you to seek out the best educational materials related to the Free Radical Therapy approach to health.

In addition to what we've already talked about, we produce books, research reports, and audio and video tapes presenting the key life-improving concepts necessary to begin enjoying improved health and vitality through Free Radical Therapy. Here are some of the currently available topics:

Mercury And Amalgam Research Reports
These 2 to 6 page reports cover political and health aspects of the mercury issue.
Porphyrin Testing, IV-C
ADA's Media Campaign

Health Realities Journal
These 8 to 12 page research reports cover one topic in great detail, telling you scientific background and methods of handling the health problems discussed.
Toxic Footprints
   Part I: Identifying, Isolating and Eliminating Chronic Bodily Toxic Contamination
   Part II: Clinical Implications of Chronic Toxic Exposure
   Part III: Iron Status: The Good, The Bad, The Ironic

Detox Essentials
   Part I: Whole Eggs—Magic Bullets
   Part II: The Mercury-binding Proteins
Protease Enzymes:
   Part I: Laying The Groundwork For Clinical Use
   Part II: Progression, Growth & Metastasis of Cancer
   Part III: Victory Over Cancer Using Trypsin
Creatine: An Investigative Report
I Thought I Was Supposed To Be Taking Vitamin C!
Things That "Bug" Us: Mercury, Rising Disease
Rates, Microbes...
Prescription For Health: Part II, Focus On The
Individual
Free Radical Therapy And The Health Model
   Part I: Free Radicals, Oxidants, And Oxidative Stress
           As A Cause Of Disease
   Part II: Antioxidants
   Part III: Inflammation
   Part IV: Acidemia And Free Calcium Excess

(see www.healthrealities.com for more titles)

Other Essential Reading
Chronic Mercury Toxicity: New Hope Against
      An Endemic Disease
This is the first medical reference book that has been written on the topic of mercury toxicity. It completely details the problem and it's treatment.
The IV-C Mercury Tox Program:
      A Guide for the Patient
This guide–a companion book for the mercury text-book–gives you a basic detoxification program that applies whether or not mercury is the source of your health problem.

Audiotapes

Health Realities in the News audio series
   These audio tapes contain interviews with Sam Queen on key health issues in the popular press and how they affect you.
Periodontal Disease/Heart Disease Connection
Antioxidant Update
Light, Cancer And Osteoporosis
Osteoporosis And Estrogen
American Heart Association Findings
Biochemical Individuality
Nitric Oxide
Pancreatic Function, Autism and pH
Weight Control – Part 1
Weight Control – Part 2
Metal Poisoning: Sources & Detection
Challenge Tests To Assess Heavy Metal Burden
Protease Enzymes: Their Impact On Your Health
Protease Enzymes: Who Is A Candidate?
Free Iron – Part 1
Free Iron – Part 2
Natural Ways To Fight Cancer – Part 1
Natural Ways To Fight Cancer – Part 2
How To Find Reality In Health News
You're Diagnosed With Cancer: Now What?
Soy: Dangerous Or Healthy Food?
Stem Cells: Panacea Or The Making of a Beast
BioTerrorism: You Can Prepare To Survive – Part 1
BioTerrorism: You Can Prepare To Survive – Part 2

Rebuilding Your Patient's Health Through Free Radical Therapy
   The most detailed available information on understanding and using Free Radical Therapy. Meant for the health professional, but also used by individuals

who are ready to learn options for improving their own health. Eight audiocassettes in an album with an accompanying booklet. Also includes the 4 printed research reports on Free Radical Therapy.

Videotapes
Administering Intravenous Vitamin C
Super Symposium 2000

Put Down the Duckie Newsletter
Put Down The Duckie is an easy-to-understand newsletter that helps you to make healthy changes gradually. It takes you through one relatively simple aspect of health at a time, giving you background information on why it's important to do, suggestions on how to work it into your lifestyle, tips, recipes and encouragement!

Changing Habits: Adding Lemon to Your Water
Butter Wars: Using Butter Instead of Margarine
Use It, Don't Lose It: Getting Enough Protein
Against the Grain: Switching to Whole Wheat
Do Something ...Anything: Beginning to Exercise
Organically Speaking: Using Organic Dairy Products
How Sweet It Is...Or Is It? Avoiding White Sugar
Sugar: Choosing Substitutes
What's On Tap? Drinking Water
Fear of Frying: Using the Best Oils for Your Health
     See *www.putdowntheduckie.com* for more information or to subscribe.

Getting More Information
     If you'd like to know more about any of these resources, please call us at (719) 598-4968, or connect to our web site at *http://www.healthrealties.com*.

Chapter Four: Generic vs. Specific Health Plans
What The Six Subclinical Areas Mean To You

The Generic Approach

Generic has some merit.

It allows someone on a limited budget to enjoy a wider variety of activities and products. We also believe there is some merit in the generic advice health authorities give to the "average" person (whoever that is), to eat a balanced diet, get plenty of exercise, watch your weight, don't smoke, and engage in some meaningful activity. On the other hand, generic health approaches fail to address individual needs, and the fact that you are biochemically unique.

Our Usual Regimen

While our main goal is to uncover ways to individualize health programs, the diet we most often lean toward can be described as a modified ovo-lacto-vegetarian diet. We recommend the routine use of fresh lemon added to drinking water, and supplementation with vitamins E and C, garlic oil, and "friendly bacteria," among other things.

Our standard diet and supplementation regimens are good starting points, but they do not address the unique needs of specific individuals. For instance, some people have an overload of body iron, or evidence of general acidity with calcium oxalate in the urine. In these cases, we would have to immediately amend the "usual" diet and supplement program. Since there are so many other possible examples, a personal health evaluation is really the only way to go, if optimum health is what you seek.

Getting Specific About Personal Evaluations

If you want to obtain our help in individualizing your program (through a consultation based on your blood chemistry) you begin by joining our Health Connection Action Group.

Time and resource constraints require us to limit the availability of consultations to those who are Action Group members. When you join you receive essential background information on Free Radical Therapy and the related Health Model. Becoming familiar with this approach before seeking personalized help enables Action Group members to make maximum gain.

Our personal health evaluations are all based upon the six fundamental subclinical defects described earlier. Identifying these defect areas, subclassifying them further, and considering them in light of blood and urine chemistry results, allows us to individualize a program of diet, supplementation and lifestyle. As a result, our evaluations are truly tailored to the unique needs of the individual.

This "tailoring" concept is not a new idea. It has been promoted before by many would-be health consultants. Approaches which are not based on the Free Radical Therapy concept, however, are unlikely to prove effective, even when total nutrient status is considered. This is the basic reason behind the failure of these programs. For success, what's called for is a comprehensive approach that keeps in mind the patterns of health interaction and the requirements of Free Radical Therapy as determined by the Health Model.

Why Individualized Evaluations Are Necessary

Have you ever pushed in on a large balloon? Wherever you pushed in, some other part of the balloon "bulged" out. Dealing with individual health is a lot like this. What we change in one area affects all the rest.

Failure to adequately address this health reality is one of the principle shortcomings of most medical and dental treatments today.

As we've said before, the currently accepted Disease Model of today's standard of care forces doctors to focus on the treatment of symptoms and risk factors. Again, treating the symptoms and addressing risk factors has some merit, but fails to get at the cause. Rather than dealing with the individual's health needs as a whole, this approach is much like pushing on a balloon.

Addressing defects in the six subclinical areas requires dealing with them in a particular order as determined by your individual circumstances. If this truth is ignored, even those familiar with Free Radical Therapy's Health Model are likely to end up pushing on the balloon. Taking this approach may result in unwanted health "bulges."

The following discussion is merely a starting point. Our aim is to provide you with enough information to get you thinking. Treatment plans, however, should be based upon comprehensive evaluations of the relevant chemistries, lifestyle and diet data by those thoroughly familiar with Free Radical Therapy and the underlying Health Model.

With this in mind...

What Does Subclinical Mean?

'Subclinical' is the term applied to conditions, symptoms and measurements which are not readily visible, and not commonly associated with a given diagnosis.

For instance, people who have an infection with fever readily recognize both of those realities, but the subclinical signs that the diagnostician might use to confirm this fact would be the presence of acid stress and chronic inflammation. Going further, body temperatures above 100° are usually considered evidence of a fever. 'Fever' is the common description given to an unseen, subclinical inflammatory response indicated by the clinical result measured by the thermometer. Again, fever is the clinical sign. Inflammation is mostly subclinical. You can solve the fever with aspirin, but that doesn't address the cause. Identifying inflammation (and acid stress) and determining the cause of each is fundamental to providing a lasting solution to the problem which we refer to as a "fever."

Looking at temperature in another way, a drop in temperature of two to four tenths of a degree (from 98.4° to 98.2°) is not generally considered an indicator of any specific clinical result. This small temperature deviation–while measurable–is not currently considered a part of any clinical condition to which a label can be applied. Does this mean that subclinical measurements and observations cannot be indicators of disease, or the beginning of some process that may lead to disease? We have a client whose family showed us that (for them) this was an important subclinical sign of things to come.

The client and his family claimed that just prior to coming down with sinus infections they all ran a slightly negative temperature. For that family, two-tenths of a degree below normal was a significant indicator of impending sinus infection. Thus, data that at first might appear to be within normal limits–but which lies either at the high or low end of normal–may actually signal some subclinical event that will soon lead to a clinical event. Subclinical changes, then, can occur and be detected in measurable body parameters, which (when fully understood) can help bring about a more meaningful treatment approach to the subclinical areas of Free Radical Therapy.

Following are the six fundamental subclinical areas. Defects in these areas are meaningful. All disease is signaled by the onset of these conditions.

1. Acid Stress

Acid stress is a drop in pH below normal, which causes a number of negative health effects. Acid stress and anaerobic conditions (i.e., lack of oxygen) go hand in hand, providing the best possible growing conditions for most disease-causing bacteria and yeast. Acid stress further harms your health by lowering your tolerance to heavy metals and other oxidant catalysts. It predisposes to calcium deposits and free calcium excess, and promotes a wide range of disease conditions.

Working past the technical jargon, acid stress opposes health by promoting conditions conducive to heart disease, osteoporosis, arthritis and cancer. In addition, acid stress promotes free calcium excess (another subclinical defect).

How is acid stress determined?

You'll probably recall from high school chemistry that pH is the measure of acidity versus alkalinity (or "baseness") of a solution. The scale runs from 0 to 14 with 7 representing neutrality. Numbers below 7 indicate increasing degrees of acidity while numbers greater than 7 measure increasing alkalinity.

The human body contains a number of fluids whose pH values are key parameters. The most commonly used are the pH of arterial blood, extra cellular fluid (ECF), urine and saliva.

Ideal arterial and ECF pH is 7.4 while 7.0 is the ideal pH for saliva. For urine, pH may rise and fall healthfully between pH 5.5-7.0, but when there is evidence of subclinical defects or risk of infection, ideal is around 7.0.

Acid stress is indicated if your pH readings fall below the ideals noted above. Infrequently, the opposite of acid stress (alkalinity) occurs. Alkalinity is seen when pH exceeds the ideal values noted above. Excessive alkalinity can bring about the same anaerobic conditions as acid stress, but it is much more rare.

You can do a simple test for acid stress by using Hydrion pH Test Papers.

The test uses a pH-sensitive, color-matched test strip. (Hydrion test strips are what we prefer. Hydrazine test strips are an acceptable alternative–but are less stable and can give variable results). You dip a test strip into urine or wet it with saliva. pH is determined by comparing the color within 30 seconds with the color chart provided with the pH test strips. An acid pH reading of saliva is a reliable indicator of acid stress, regardless of the urine pH. The urine pH is nevertheless helpful, especially if you're dealing with a urinary tract infection or yeast infection. In this situation, every effort must be made to bring the urine pH to neutral or slightly alkaline.

If you're interested in self-testing, you can obtain Hydrion pH paper by contacting us.

2. Anaerobic Tendency

An anaerobic tendency means the body is operating more in anaerobic metabolism and less in aerobic metabolism than is optimal. *Anaerobic* means living in the absence of oxygen. *Aerobic* means living in the presence of oxygen. The body is operating both aerobically and anaerobically all of the time.

In aerobic metabolism, the body produces 36 ATP energy molecules for each molecule of glucose burned. In anaerobic metabolism, the body only produces 2 ATP energy molecules per molecule of glucose burned. It's easy to see that you'll have less energy if you have an anaerobic tendency.

It's important to deal with a tendency towards anaerobic metabolism because of its negative health effects. Anaerobic metabolism leads to gingivitis, yeast infections, periodontitis, persistent bacterial infections and tooth decay. It can predispose you to diabetes, arterial disease, cancer, fatigue and all degenerative processes.

Chronic anaerobic metabolism can be caused by a number of factors including acid stress, diabetes, glucose intolerance and/or high blood sugar, a deficiency in vitamin C, overeating, lack of physical exercise, failure to eat complete dietary proteins, anemia, excess phosphate, lung disease, and chronic infections. A blood chemistry analysis can determine the causes of anaerobic metabolism.

Blood work can also determine whether you have a low-energy or high-energy type of anaerobic tendency. Either type can lead to fatigue, but they are handled differently.

3. Free Calcium Excess

Free calcium excess is the result of chronic acid stress, and the most consistent indicator of altered pH. In cases where a saliva pH has not been performed, an excess of free calcium noted on the blood chemistry profile is a strong predictor of an acid saliva pH of ≤ 6.5.

So, what is free calcium excess?

The calcium that circulates in the blood is comprised

of both bound calcium (55% of the total) and free cal-cium (45% of the total). Bound calcium is bound either to protein or to an alkaline buffer. When either protein is low or alkaline buffers are inadequate, then the percentage of free calcium rises. Thus, as free calcium rises above normal there is naturally a drop in pH.

A normal level of free calcium (45% of total) is essential to life, as it helps activate nearly every body process. So it is healthy to have free calcium. However, excesses of free calcium (when free calcium makes up 47-49% of the total), caused by either a drop in consumption of protein or alkaline buffers, can lead to calcium deposits and a wide variety of health problems. These range from calculus on the teeth to calcified arteries and high blood pressure. Fundamentally, then, these and many other problems may result from a deficiency of protein and/or a reduction in alkaline buffer. Since phosphate is the primary alkaline buffer, the delicate "teeter-totter" effect of bound vs. free calcium can be estimated by looking at the ratio of calcium to phosphorous. In people with adequate protein intake, serum calcium levels which exceed a 2.5 to 1 ratio with the phosphate reading tend to accurately reflect free calcium excess. (We mention this to give you an example of how laboratory data assists in evaluating your health status.)

As indicated previously, the excess free calcium is then available for a host of health problems. In addition to calculus and calcified arteries, it may lead to arthritis, gall stones, kidney stones, and high blood pressure. Excess free calcium can also stimulate chronic inflammation. By bringing about an anaerobic tendency, free calcium excess is connected with cancer. Breast cancer, for instance, is often identified by looking for signs of calcification on the X-ray.

Controlling acid stress is a routine first step in overcoming free calcium excess, and in thereby reducing the risk of many health conditions. Adequate dietary intake of phosphorous rich foods such as eggs, nuts, and seeds (especially pumpkin seeds), is a good step. After this, however, it gets more complicated. In our seminar series for doctors, they're instructed in how to identify and respond to a seven-layered buffering system. What we've described here relates to only one of those layers. The total approach is more complex, yet easily learned by those with health backgrounds.

The necessary testing to adequately evaluate free calcium excess and all seven of the buffering layers includes the required blood, urine, and saliva tests along with the related lifestyle and diet data.

There are no easy procedures which just anyone can perform here. It's going to take a blood chemistry evaluation. So, obviously, the cooperation of your doctor is required from this point forward. Toward this end, we recommend the services of those thoroughly trained in Free Radical Therapy and the underlying Health Model.

If your doctor is not familiar with the Free Radical Therapy concept, membership in the Action Group can help put you in touch with health practitioners who are.

4. Chronic Inflammation

The term "inflammation" is often thought of as a pathological event. Yet, by design, inflammation is a perfectly normal, health-promoting occurrence. It's how your body is designed to repair itself, fight infections, deal with toxic exposures, and fight cancer successfully. Nevertheless, if your body does not have what it needs to bring the inflammatory response to a successful close, then chronic inflammation sets in.

Unlike the healthy inflammatory response, chronic

inflammation is connected with virtually every disease in which the immune system is compromised. Chronic inflammation is also connected with virtually all chronic diseases (including coronary artery disease, coronary thrombosis, heart attack, cancer, arthritis, and stroke).

Again, it is essential to recognize that inflammation in and of itself is not a bad thing: It is a good thing "gone awry," causing chronic inflammation.

Chronic inflammation is bad because:

- It produces enzymes that attack and destroy connective tissues, thereby bringing about aging and disease due to a breakdown of all cells and organs. Arterial narrowing, fibromyalgia, and loose teeth are all linked to this fundamental, subclinical defect.
- It dilutes any attempt to fight infections. Chronic sinus infections and the conversion of HIV positive to the onset of AIDS are both encouraged by chronic inflammation.
- It impairs the mix of lymphocytes necessary in our cancer defense system. Ovarian cancer, for instance, often follows many years of ovarian cysts driven by chronic inflammation where the body gives up fighting the toxins involved in cyst formation.
- It is the most significant source of free radicals. Free radicals further destroy connective tissues and other cell parts as well, and are thereby associated with virtually all degenerative conditions including aging and cancer.
- It stimulates antibody production that makes worse all autoimmune conditions, such as Lupus, multiple sclerosis, rheumatoid arthritis, diabetes, and Sjøgren's disease.

Anti-inflammatory drugs do a great job in rescuing– but eventually fail. The exciting part is that in many cases, diet and supplementation can effectively take over. They do this by supporting the body's design to correct chronic inflammation naturally.

An Extraordinary Example

The most dramatic case we've seen corrected by this approach involved a 22-year-old woman who had been diagnosed with chronic autoimmune hepatitis. Her body built antibodies against the connective tissues of her liver. As a result, her immune system began treating her liver as if it were an invading, foreign entity. Her doctor rescued her with Prednisone. Unfortunately, the continued use of Prednisone began leading to unwanted side effects. This required him to reduce the dosage or risk unrelated damage. Then, since the doctor could not halt the production of antibodies, the young woman became a candidate for a liver transplant. At this point, her doctor incorporated the Free Radical Therapy approach.

Three years later her liver enzyme readings were restored to normal and she was able to handle her problem without Prednisone. To our knowledge she is the only person with this condition to escape the liver transplant route without dying.

Free Radical Therapy Doctors And
HealthConnection Reports

If you're interested in combating chronic inflammation through our methods, we encourage you to contact a doctor who is familiar with our methods, or to arrange a comprehensive, HealthConnection written report through our office. This evaluation is done for your unique health situation and is based on key blood and urine indices along with related lifestyle and diet data, and an oral health assessment.

The written HealthConnection report is essentially a report all about your own health. It archives your health status at a given point in time, and provides a detailed explanation regarding your health status as it relates to our Health Model approach. The report ends with an action program giving the steps necessary for you and your doctor to apply the appropriate Free Radical Therapy regimen to your specific health needs. In addition—once you receive your report—a half hour individual consultation is scheduled in order to make certain that you understand your health needs from the Free Radical Therapy perspective.

5. Connective Tissue Breakdown

Before explaining how connective tissue breakdown contributes to aging and disease, let's first explain its makeup and purpose.

Visualize a large skyscraper in downtown Manhattan. Before such a building could become so tall and stable, the engineers first installed a superstructure of steel and concrete. In your body, this superstructure is composed of bone. Yet, unlike a skyscraper, your body must be flexible, so the bone is broken up into many sections. To tie the bony sections together and give your body flexibility, guywire-like substances (ligaments and tendons) are used. These represent one type of connective tissue. To tie these to other cells and organs, supportive cytoplasmic elements are added. They're designed not only for attachment, but also to provide integrity to cells or to organize intracellular organelles, or compartments. Some connective tissues tie the cells in place, while still others serve to separate one organ from another. In addition, connective tissue (such as cartilage) may give flexibility and strength to joints.

All connective tissues are made from a protein-rich collagen and a carbohydrate-rich proteoglycan lattice. By attachment of the collagen proteins to the lattice-like structure, a wide variety of connective tissues can be synthesized to match whatever tensile strength and function is required.

The problem is that chronic inflammation, instead of building connective tissue (as is the intention of the healthful inflammatory response), begins producing enzymes that destroy connective tissue. In other cases your body builds antibodies against the protein aspect of the connective tissues.

As connective tissue weakens from this action, what happens next?

Many health problems begin to appear, starting with compromised oral health. Your gums develop a tendency towards bleeding when you floss or brush, your gum line begins receding, and your teeth become loose. Elsewhere, you may bruise easily, and develop varicose veins, hemorrhoids, or weak back muscles. Hiatal hernias and aneurysms may follow. Tissues may sag. This is especially true around the facial area where connective tissues must necessarily have less tensile strength (allowing the movement necessary for speech and facial expressions). It also occurs in the breast, the abdomen, and all the other unwanted areas we so painfully become aware of as we get older!

When you overcome the problem of connective tissue breakdown, then, you not only end up healthier, but can also look better. And with all the money you can spend on appearance-enhancing products, this is a pretty inexpensive and effective way to accomplish that with the additional benefit of improved health.

How do we stop connective tissue breakdown, and how do we rebuild tissues?

You must first handle chronic inflammation, which may require also handling acid stress and free calcium excess. Since connective tissue may be destroyed by

the free radical by-products of oxidative stress, then
oxidative stress must also be handled. After that, you
need to consume adequate protein and add to your diet
supplements that are specific to rebuilding connective
tissues.

In theory, if you could eliminate connective tissue
breakdown entirely, you would be on your way to stop-
ping (or perhaps even reversing) the aging process.
When all the answers are available to accomplish this,
you will find that Free Radical Therapy offers the con-
ceptual framework for implementing the required steps.
Ultimately, the appropriate practice of the Free Radical
Therapy concepts aids our ability to correctly apply these
new findings as they become available.

A further advantage to having the required concep-
tual framework already in place is that you don't have
to wait for all the answers to be in. By employing the
available Free Radical Therapy concepts now, you can
begin to reduce the ravages of connective tissue breakdown.

6. Oxidative Stress

Oxidative stress is the unhealthy accumulation of high
energy free radicals within human chemistries.

Oxidation is the primary process by which humans
and higher animals derive sufficient energy to be mo-
bile. It is the consequence of oxygen reacting electro-
chemically with some oxidant catalyst, such as iron.
Such reactions release a high level of energy which,
when controlled, keeps you healthy, active, and strong.

From body-produced oxidation there arises a boun-
tiful quantity of controlled energy. Along with this benefit, there is a potential source of uncontrolled energy—
a chemical species that has an unpaired set of electrons
in its outer orbit. This by-product, commonly known as

a free radical, is used by the body to stimulate some healthful events (such as the killing of bacteria, or the eventual excretion of fat-soluble toxins), but when present in excess a host of unhealthful events may take place. Any excess of free radicals may lead to destruction of cellular components, including the alteration of DNA and RNA.

In health, your body is designed to control the energy from oxidation and to maintain a healthful balance of the free radical by-products. An imbalance often occurs due either to a lack of antioxidants or to excessive exposure to oxidant catalysts. These may include certain toxic heavy metals, particularly mercury, lead, arsenic, tin, and cadmium. An excess of oxidant catalysts may also arise from otherwise health-promoting metals, such as copper and iron. Other oxidant catalysts include the many chemicals, solvents, and pesticides mentioned earlier in this book. As noted previously, they are a consequence of our environment being contaminated from their overuse in industry and medicine. Severe and sometimes irreparable damage can result from these exposures.

Many of the chemicals, pesticides, organic solvents, and toxic metals have a deleterious effect on the brain and nerves. Thus, as you might expect, prolonged oxidative stress often results in nerve and brain disorders. Excess iron and exposure to pesticides, for instance, has been credited to the onset of Parkinson's disease. Exposure to mercury and a variety of other metals has been connected with Alzheimer's disease, and the list goes on. Oxidative stress is also related to free radical-induced arteriosclerosis and colon cancer. Studies reported in recent years at the American Heart Association, for instance, have connected mercury and iron exposure to heart disease. In addition, excessive exposure to oxidant catalysts and the free radicals they produce has been linked to the onset and progression of autoimmune disease. So there is good reason to include in any health program steps to eliminate oxidative stress.

Through Free Radical Therapy, much can be done to support a healthy oxidative process which adequately disposes of free radicals.

If you did nothing more than eliminate acid stress, you would be helping yourself immensely towards reducing oxidative stress. Free radicals are produced far more abundantly in an acid environment than in a neutral or alkaline environment. Lemon juice, apple juice, seeds, zinc and magnesium aid in this process, because they help eliminate acid and control pH. Cultured dairy foods and foods rich in monounsaturated fatty acids (i.e., most soaked, raw nuts) are also key. All of these either provide a better balance in pH, or supply antioxidants (directly or indirectly). Another important measure would be to eat enough protein, which binds to oxidant catalysts and helps neutralize them. Having an adequate copper level is also helpful, since copper helps in selectively distributing energy to the more tender tissues that would be destroyed if iron were the energy transport metal.

Oxidative stress is a growing problem that often requires specific supplementation along with appropriate diet and lifestyle adjustments.

Efforts to control it by simply supplementing with antioxidants very often fail. This is because antioxidants themselves can be oxidized to a free radical entity. To avoid this mistake, doctors are advised to make specific adjustments.

Such adjustments are readily identified through a thorough and properly prepared Free Radical Therapy evaluation as can be obtained by the HealthConnection analysis or consultation.

How The Six Subclinical Areas Relate To Genetics, Disease, And Health

Genetics and the so-called "gene pool" that you get from your parents are the driving forces behind what makes you different. Similarly, genetics will make a difference to your susceptibility or resistance to the six subclinical defects that precede and/or accompany disease. Your body draws upon its strong points, and for every weakness, has a compensatory mechanism. A good example of this is the seven levels to the buffering system. Even if one of those areas is defective, the other six are sufficient to control pH as long as you understand what is required. That, and the fact that each of us has varying capacities to overcome toxic exposure and exposure to potential pathogens, provides evidence for the need to take into account biochemical individuality. Personalized evaluations better predict and control the effectiveness of each push we give to the "balloon" and thereby how to more effectively correct the six fundamental defects.

There is, however, a sequence to our approach. Obviously, life-threatening conditions must be dealt with first.

Once your health is stabilized, optimum results are obtained only by addressing the six subclinical areas in a particular order. Free calcium excess is more easily remedied, for instance, if you begin with the handling of acid stress.

Similarly, chronic inflammation is less problematic and more readily responds to effort when acid stress and free calcium excess are handled first. This is why so many failures are encountered by doctors who mistakenly believe they are offering Free Radical Therapy (a health model-based approach) when they begin their programs with antioxidant therapy (a non-comprehensive approach).

It is essential to keep in mind that the major antioxidants, such as vitamins C, E, and beta carotene, work by donating electrons–a function that is greatly slowed in an acidic environment. Couple this with the fact that oxidant catalysts produce free radicals at a faster rate in an acidic environment and you can see that failure to overcome acid stress first is an illogical approach. In addition,, once an antioxidant has donated its electrons it becomes another oxidized entity that is capable of causing damage, and must therefore be reduced back to its original state by another antioxidant.

Again, this process is slowed by an acidic environment, which accounts for why supplementing with too-low doses of antioxidants may actually cause more harm than good. The effect of this could be seen in the Finnish study reported just several years ago in a leading journal, in which smokers who were supplemented with low doses of antioxidants tended to develop more lung cancer than smokers who received no supplementation.

Again, appropriate attention to these six subclinical areas within the framework of the Health Model tends to generate very favorable results, while administering the program 'helter-skelter' gives unpredictable results. This is another advantage of obtaining a HealthConnection report or consultation before starting your program, or in soliciting the help of a doctor beforehand who has been thoroughly trained in Free Radical Therapy.

Chapter Five: The Basic Diet
One Diet Does Not Work For All

One size fits all is a nice idea, but if you've ever tried one on, you know the concept doesn't work all that well! This tends to be true as well in both diet and food supplementation. It's the basic flaw behind public health-driven programs, in which you're advised to be immunized, go on a low-fat/low-cholesterol diet, and get all the nutrients you need by eating a so-called "balanced" diet that contains the recommended daily allowance (RDA) for each nutrient. Such programs fit a few people nicely, but some react adversely to immunizations, and others die as a result of eating low-fat/low-cholesterol "everything". No one knows for certain just what a balanced diet really is, and it is difficult to accurately determine just how much of any nutrient is present in the food we eat.

Thus, just as taking measurements for clothing is fundamental to obtaining the correct fit, optimum health poses different requirements for each of us due to the uniqueness of our specific needs. For this reason it's essential to analyze key blood and urine factors, a dental assessment, and your dietary and lifestyle patterns before providing individual recommendations. Keep this in mind as you read on. We'll outline for you our general dietary recommendations, but without knowing your specific health situation, these may not be enough. Following them will, however, almost certainly improve most people's health to some degree.

The Modified Ovo-Lacto-Vegetarian Diet

Our diet can generally be described as a modified ovo-lacto-vegetarian diet.

Ovo refers to eggs. Contrary to the negative press

given cholesterol, eggs are an essential part of both detoxification and a healthy diet. Further, by stimulating the production of apoprotein E, eggs will generally aid in the moderation of healthy cholesterol levels. This is particularly true if you have good bowel function, exercise regularly, take vitamin C supplements, and eat a high fiber diet.

Lacto means the lactase-rich foods, such as yogurt, soft cheeses, and other cultured dairy products. It does <u>not</u> include milk. Plain, unsweetened yogurt, which may be eaten "as is" or with the addition of strawberries or raw sunflower seeds, is an important part of your daily diet. If you are lactose intolerant, further modification is necessary, but it is all worth the effort. Overcoming lactose intolerance and the perceived problem of forming mucus (which <u>can</u> be done) is fundamental to successful detoxification and getting off the antibiotic treadmill.

Vegetarian is self-explanatory. Keep in mind, however, that this diet is "modified." It's modified in the sense that we recommend the inclusion of organically fed poultry and lamb along with Alaskan salmon. The *vegan*, or strict vegetarian diet, often does not provide adequate protein since vegetable protein by itself is insufficient in people with significant contaminant exposures. However, with the addition of poultry, lamb, salmon, eggs, cultured dairy foods, and a few other foods, you've got what it takes to overcome toxicity.

The Big Protein Breakfast

We like to see a "big protein" breakfast. Typically, this means two eggs and/or a good serving of natural, whole grain cereal. If you're sensitive to these foods, there are alternatives at first, and then there are ways of overcoming the sensitivities.

Along with eggs and whole grains, nuts and seeds are also good protein sources. We recommend raw pumpkin seeds and sunflower seeds, eaten whole or blended in a mixer with natural apple juice and (perhaps) some yogurt or protein supplement (to which can be added a few drops of vanilla for flavor, if you want). The seeds are particularly beneficial when eaten with plain, unsweetened yogurt. If you prefer flavor to your yogurt, be aware of the sugar additives in many fruited yogurts. A better choice is to add fresh strawberries or red grapes to plain, unsweetened yogurt. (Some fruits can thwart your attempts at improving health, so it's better to learn more about them before adding just any fruit. This is another reason why we can only give you general diet recommendations without a complete health evaluation.)

Things to Avoid in Your Diet

Milk is discouraged in this program, as are refined carbohydrates. Refined carbohydrates include things made with refined sugar and white, processed flours, such as donuts, bagels, or croissants. Also to be discouraged are coffee, carbonated beverages preserved with phosphoric acid, and most red meats.

Corn, potatoes, orange juice and bananas are discouraged due to their high sugar content. A whole orange on occasion is acceptable. Keep in mind, however, that we are trying to counter acid stress. Consequently, too many simple sugars may cause a loss in the urine of alkaline buffers, particularly phosphate and magnesium.

An occasional grapefruit and/or a small glass of grapefruit juice is okay. Apple juice, apple cider, and even apple cider vinegar are recommended for pH control since these foods all stimulate the pancreas to dump bicarbonate buffer into the small intestines. This causes the whole body to become more alkaline.

Working with Whole Grains

There are some wonderful natural whole grain cereals available. We recommend our recipe included in this book's appendix. It's inexpensive, easy to make, and delicious. Our "egg cocktail"–also included–can be used in place of milk on the whole grain cereal. Those who prefer something else are encouraged to use cultured milk products such as liquid yogurt. If you can't live without milk, then we recommend at least minimizing the quantity of milk you consume, and using acidophilus milk in place of your regular kind. Acidophilus milk is available in health food stores and in many of the larger grocery chains. The difference in taste is so minor you may not even notice it. Be careful with the amount of rice milk you consume since it is generally very rich in carbohydrates.

Many of the people contacting our office are either sensitive to gluten in wheat, or are afflicted with an autoimmune or inflammatory disorder. If you have any of these problems you should avoid gluten-containing grains. You would do better to resort to brown rice, millet, and spelt.

Those requiring a tighter dietary approach will do better following our recipe for homemade whole grain cereal. For flavor and variety, it can't be beat!

Whole Grain Flours

We should also briefly mention that cooking with whole grain flours is a different world compared to cooking with the refined white, bleached flours most of America uses. There are a lot of different whole grain flours readily available in the specialty foods sections of most grocery and health food stores. These include whole wheat, oat, barley, rye, and amaranth (to mention a few).

Each of these flours has its own cooking properties. The whole grain flours are all much "heavier" than refined white flours. Also, most of the whole grain flours are less "glue-like" than the refined white variety. Your cooking results will tend to be more crumbly. As you become a "gourmet" health food chef, you will learn to make adjustments in recipes. In the meantime, none of us has suffered from simply substituting whole grain flour in the same proportion as the white flour called for in recipes! We actually now prefer the improved texture and taste of the whole grain product.

Major manufacturers and establishments often mix white flour in with the whole grain flour to produce a product that they think the public will eat. You need to be aware of this when eating out or purchasing something that says "whole wheat."

If you can't get used to the whole grain texture, you might want to add a little unbleached, *organic* white flour (remembering that even though it's organic, white flour can still contribute to acid stress). Another option is to use whole wheat pastry flour, which in some recipes produces a lighter product. You can also substitute unsweetened applesauce for up to 1/2 cup of the fat called for in a recipe, which also results in a lighter (and healthier) product.

For more information on grains and other foods, see our *Put Down the Duckie* newsletter.

Raw Honey: The Sweetener Of Choice

A word about honey is now in order: Not all honeys that say "natural" are actually so. This is true even when they are clearly marked "100 percent honey" on their labels. Major processors of honey often heat their product. This serves two purposes. It reduces the enzyme activity, which helps stabilize the flavor, and it kills the spore that may cause botulism in children under one year of age. In addition, the manufacturer may add sugar or corn syrup to keep it from crystallizing in the winter. These alterations seem harmless enough, but in reality they greatly reduce health value. In adults, the real stuff is capable of resisting the growth of nearly every organism that causes disease, and it nourishes the friendly bacteria by supplying a healthy dose of fructooligosaccharide, which is also referred to as FOS.

Another healthy sweetener is stevia, which is available in most health foods stores.

Following Biblical Nutrition

For those of you who want to know what the Bible has to say about health, you may be interested in Isaiah's prophecy of what Jesus would eat as a youngster. In Isaiah 7: 15, *"Butter* (translated in Hebrew as a yogurt-like drink) and *honey* shall He eat, that He may know the good and resist the evil."

This keeps shepherds of the Mideast region free of disease today just as it did 2,000 years ago, and has the potential of doing the same for you. Not only does it help prevent infections, but regular consumption of cultured dairy foods and raw honey represents one of the most effective means known today for detoxification.

The best place to find raw, natural honey that has not been adulterated with heat or sugar is through your local beekeeper. If there are no beekeepers in your vicinity that sell directly to the public, then check with your local health food store.

Fresh Lemon Juice: Overcoming Acid Stress

We encourage the routine consumption of fresh lemon

juice throughout the day and particularly first thing in the morning. Fresh lemons are preferred, but when in a hurry, Minute Maid™ produces a fresh frozen lemon juice that is also acceptable and can be found in the frozen food section of grocery stores. (For emphasis, we are recommending *fresh* lemon juice which has been frozen. We are not talking about the unfrozen lemon juice found on grocery shelves since it contains a pre-servative.)

We suggest mixing one to two tablespoons of fresh lemon juice in cold or hot water, without sugar or other sweeteners, and drinking it first thing in the morning, and then throughout the day. If you are using a micro-wave oven to warm your water, however, heat the water first and then add the lemon juice. There is some concern that microwaving may damage food enzymes.

Fresh Fruits And Vegetables, Beans And Lentils

Fresh fruits that are encouraged include apples, straw-berries, grapes, pineapple, papaya, lemons, kiwi, and mangos.

When it comes to vegetables, we want you to know that leafy green produce, along with cultured dairy foods, are your best source of body-usable calcium. Leafy green vegetables also provide a rich source of vitamin C, and they enhance your daily fiber content.

Red and yellow vegetables are also recommended. Those vegetables which are bright in color (whether green, red, yellow, purple or orange) tend to be good sources of the carotenoid family of nutrients, which include vitamin A. Carrots are a good source of those caro-tenoids that stimulate immune function, but other rich sources of carotenoids include yams, yellow squash, kale, spinach, and red bell peppers.

Beans and lentils are excellent fiber sources and

should be included in your diet, especially if you've gotten overweight from eating too many carbohydrates relative to protein.

We Need More Garlic

Garlic is perhaps the most versatile of the detoxifying foods, for a variety of reasons. Garlic is a rich source of sulfhydryl proteins that bind to mercury and other heavy metals, and thereby help get these contaminants out of the body. Garlic also helps control the balance of the naturally-occurring intestinal bacteria. It does this by also providing FOS (a source of nutrient for the friendly bacteria which the unfriendly bacteria cannot consume). Garlic further helps in the control of unfriendly bacteria by being a source of sulfur that naturally kills potential pathogens, and helps to activate nitric oxide–a potent bacteria and yeast-fighting agent. In addition, the nitric oxide that garlic helps produce also helps with the relaxation of smooth muscle (which in turn is necessary to counter angina, asthma, high blood pressure, and Raynaud's syndrome).

Pass the Butter, Please!

What about butter or margarine?

As you may know, heart disease is lowest among the French who nationally consume higher amounts of butter. The French also consume less margarine than is consumed in America (where heart disease is more common).

The bottom line is that butter is better for detoxification. In addition, butter is far more protective against heart failure than margarine. On the other hand, margarine has the potential of raising cholesterol almost as much as butter. More to the point, margarine has the potential of making congestive heart failure worse.

Become A Healthy Reader

As noted before, we are big on reading! We want you to read the labels of everything you eat very carefully.

Most commercially available foods are loaded with sugars (particularly sucrose and corn syrup) and preservatives (including nitrites). Limit the intake of these foods, and avoid them wherever possible. When a product is labelled "whole wheat" or "wheat," check the ingredients. Only if it says "100% whole wheat" are you getting the whole grain product–and even then, many commercial products are still full of sugar and preservatives. The longer the list of ingredients, the less likely that food item is going to be of any use to you. It goes without saying that the closer the food you buy is to its natural state, the more nutrition you'll get from it.

You Sometimes Get What You Don't Pay For!

Just a note here, on the cost of healthier food, which many people commonly object to.

Let's compare a 1 lb. loaf of "Cracked Wheat" bread from our local grocery store at 99¢, against a 2 lb. loaf of Sunflower Whole Wheat bread at $3.29 from our local health food store. The ingredients for the 99¢ loaf read "enriched flour (flour, malted barley flour, niacin, reduced iron, thiamin mononitrate [vitamin B_1], riboflavin [vitamin B_2]), water, whole wheat flour, high fructose corn syrup, wheat gluten, wheat, yeast, honey, partially hydrogenated soybean oil, salt, yeast nutrients (calcium sulfate and ammonium chloride), calcium propionate, sodium stearoyl lactylate, caramel color, mono- and diglycerides, dough conditioners (ascorbic acid and azodicarbonamide)." This bread is nearly flavorless, and very unsatisfying. You would never just eat a slice without covering it in something.

Now the ingredients for the $3.29 loaf: "stone ground 100% organic whole wheat, honey, sunflower seeds, oil, molasses, yeast, salt." This bread is full of flavor and texture, and a slice by itself is a treat.

Which would you rather feed your family if cost were not an objective?

And is the reduced cost really a bargain when you consider the (expensive) health problems that result from unhealthful eating?

Methods Of Heating Food

We noted previously that there is some concern that microwaving may destroy food enzymes–overheating by any method can damage nutritional content. On the other hand, the microwave is a great way to reheat foods. Some foods, however, appear to tolerate the heating process better than others. Keep in mind when considering your options that convenience has to be balanced against the preservation of food value. Accordingly, we recommend discretion when it comes to heating foods.

Many foods, in fact, are better for you uncooked. On the other hand, some foods require cooking to destroy unhealthy bacteria or to make them more palatable.

When you cook vegetables, we suggest stir frying or steaming in order to seal in the natural food values. Boiled vegetables lose much nutrition into the cooking water. If you do boil vegetables, then save the broth to make soup.

Cookware

Cooking utensils can be hidden sources of contaminant materials.

You can add unwanted aluminum, tin, copper, nickel, iron and a host of other metals to your food just by using cookware with surfaces that contain these materials.

Here again we see the usual problem with our American lifestyle: Convenience tends to overshadow what's best for health. Teflon™ and other slick surfaces clean up well, but they also may shed contaminants into your food. If shedding begins, discard immediately. Copper is certainly ideal for even heat distribution, but when you cook highly acidic foods in copper pots you stand the risk of getting too much copper in your diet. The same goes for drinking water that is piped to your home through copper pipes. If the water is acidic you can become contaminated with copper.

The best cookware to minimize contaminant materials is glass or Pyrex™. Ceramic and pottery cookwares are satisfactory, if they are of good quality, and have been fired sufficiently by the manufacturer. If not, the "shiny" surfaces of these materials may shed contaminant materials when they are heated.

Chapter Six
Basic Food Supplementation

Over the years much debate has accompanied the use of food supplements.

Some doctors argue that supplements just make for "expensive urine." Yet, findings in recent years of the value of supplementing with vitamins E and C are the beginning of good reasons for supplementing with a broad range of nutrients.

Properly selected food supplements can promote the body's ability to heal itself. We include in this list the right kinds of vitamins, minerals, fatty acids, and proteins. We even include a few naturally occurring hormones, such as melatonin and/or DHEA.

Food supplements can help make up for the diminished nutritional content of many of the commercially processed foods you consume. Food supplements can also help protect you against the many pesticides used in agriculture today. To a certain extent, food supplements can also make up for inadequate dietary practices. Ultimately, however, specific supplementation can help you gain better functioning in all six subclinical areas.

How Much Of What Should I Take And...When?

In health, frequently, what we thought we knew yesterday is not what we know today. This is a common problem for most health-conscious individuals–every day you can pick up the newspaper and read seemingly contradictory information! If you have access to the Internet, we encourage you to sign up for our electronic magazine. Through this, we can help you make sense of those confusing news items.

When it comes to individual health, however, the issue is one of uniqueness. We really can't tell you what specific food supplements will benefit you most without a comprehensive look at symptoms and family history, as well as key blood/urine indices, plus all relevant lifestyle and diet patterns.

In addition, when you take your supplements can be as much (or more) important than what you take or how much you take.

For those who prefer a general approach, we recommend the detoxification regimen detailed in *The IV-C Mercury Tox Program : A Guide For The Patient*. (For information on this guide, on the HealthConnection Action Group, on the HealthConnection personal evaluation, or on other products mentioned, visit our web site at *http://www.healthrealities.com,* or call us at (719) 598-4968.)

Please keep in mind, however, that the "patient" aspect of *The IV-C Mercury Tox Program* is based on the assumption that your nutritional regimen is moderated by treatment from a doctor who thoroughly understands the Free Radical Therapy approach.

With these things in mind, here are some of the food supplements which we recommend:

Vitamin C

The value of vitamin C in the diet has been rigorously evaluated. In the process of preventing scurvy (the total breakdown of connective tissue), vitamin C serves as an efficient electron donor. These donated electrons allow us to neutralize free radicals, and it is this action that makes vitamin C the most readily available antioxidant. Vitamin C serves not only to rebuild connective tissues, but also plays an equally important role in detoxification. In addition, vitamin C serves to improve carbohydrate metabolism. Amounts that exceed what is needed are readily excreted in the urine, which keeps the oxidized form from building up when there is a high body burden of metals. In addition, vitamin C serves to modulate the inflammatory response and reduce the reactivity so often noted by those who have autoimmune disorders. To illustrate, people with food sensitivities who take ultra-megadoses of vitamin C report almost immediate relief. This is also true if you have a runny nose, and take vitamin C with lemon water.

Your source of vitamin C is very important. The sources we like are ascorbic acid and sodium ascorbate. We do not recommend calcium ascorbate. The primary reason for taking vitamin C is the benefit provided by the electrons it's capable of donating. When calcium ascorbate is your source of vitamin C, you get only 1 electron per molecule. Ascorbic acid and sodium ascorbate, on the other hand, each donate 2 electrons. Being a poor electron donor is basically why vitamin C as calcium ascorbate stays longer in the bloodstream than ascorbic acid or sodium ascorbate. And, since it is electrons that are needed to scavenge for free radicals and recharge the energy molecule (NADPH), then you get cheated when your source of vitamin C is calcium ascorbate.

Yes, it is true that the measured vitamin C level remains elevated longer with calcium ascorbate than with ascorbic acid or sodium ascorbate. This further proves that calcium ascorbate just isn't doing the job you want your vitamin C to do. If it were donating the electrons you want, then the serum level would fall much quicker (as it does following administration of ascorbic acid). Also, if further analysis of serum vitamin C could be done, you would find that what you were measuring was not the superior, reduced form of vitamin C. Instead, with calcium ascorbate, you are measuring the oxidized, free radical-like form of vitamin C. While oxidized vitamin C does provide some benefit, such as in the prevention of scurvy, it still has a number of characteristics that are self defeating. Oxidized vitamin C, for instance, has no ability to convert oxidized vitamin E to its useful, reduced state. As mentioned before, oxidized vitamin C has no electrons to donate in the scavenging of free radicals.

Beyond being a poor electron donor, vitamin C in its calcium ascorbate state adds an additional 124 mg of free calcium per 1 gram of vitamin C consumed. This makes calcium ascorbate a potential source of excess free calcium, and (thereby) a potential cause of calcification.

As for calcium ascorbate's benefit as a buffered form of C, you can get the same ascorbic acid buffering action from lemon water. Lemon juice stimulates the pancreas to release bicarbonate into the small intestines (via secretin hormone released from the duodenum). This effectively raises the pH, not only of the small intestines, but also of the saliva and urine. In addition, the citrate that gets absorbed into the bloodstream further helps raise body pH by getting involved in what biochemists refer to as the citric acid cycle.

In consideration of all these things, our maintenance dosage of vitamin C is 2 grams daily. We recommend that 2 grams be taken first thing in the morning with lemon water.

Bioflavonoids

Bioflavonoids are found in fruits and vegetables, and can be taken as a supplement. Bioflavonoids offer a unique reservoir of electrons and are a protector of Vitamin C (helps maintain Vitamin C in its reduced state).

Bioflavonoids are also useful for building connective tissues.

It's good to take bioflavonoids on an empty stomach with your Vitamin C. If you take bioflavonoids with food, it tends to act as fiber.

Vitamin E

Vitamin E modulates the inflammatory response by keeping it from occurring too rapidly. Vitamin E slows the release of aracadonic acid (from fat storage), the initiator of the inflammatory response. This also helps prevent unwanted blood clots. Vitamin E also modulates free radicals.

The form of vitamin E should be d-alpha tocopherol with mixed tocopherols such as beta, delta and gamma tocopherols. Forms such as "dl-alpha tocopheryl succinate" or acctate are all synthetic, and are not as effective. For example, gamma tocopherols are specifically needed for the neutralization of certain free radicals that cause inflammation, but it is never present in synthetic vitamin E.

We recommend taking vitamin E, blackcurrant seed oil and salmon oil at different meals, since these oils compete for absorption.

Garlic Oil

Raw garlic is nature's antibiotic. It helps relax smooth muscle throughout the body, and the sulfhydryl proteins it contains helps to remove mercury and other toxic metals.

Those of us who had parents or grandparents who gave us raw garlic when we were children are discovering new wisdom in those old wives' tales. While raw garlic is about as easy to take as cod liver oil (which we don't recommend for adults), there are alternatives.

Garlic oil capsules are much easier to ingest, and possess all the properties we expect from raw garlic in detoxification. In addition, there are more socially accepted, odorless forms for those who do not wish to become "socially challenged." (Let garlic cloud your breath in company and you'll know what we are talking about!)

Blackcurrant Seed Oil

Blackcurrant seed oil is one of the best sources of naturally occurring gamma linolenic acid (GLA). Gamma linolenic acid is essential for making the Series 1 Prostaglandin hormones needed to shut inflammation down healthfully. In addition, GLA is oxidized to di-homo-linolenic acid (DGLA). Di-homo-linolenic acid competes with arachidonic acid for oxidizing enzymes and thereby helps reduce the risk of unwanted thrombus, or blood clots.

As a result, blackcurrant seed oil is fundamental in overcoming chronic inflammation.

Salmon Oil (or a distilled, Nordic fish oil)

Salmon oil is the most concentrated source of omega 3 fatty acids. Omega 3 fatty acids benefit the inflammatory response through their involvement in the synthesis of the Series 3 prostaglandin hormones. In addition, omega 3's help prevent thrombus formation by slowing the conversion of arachidonic acid to the leukotrienes involved in clot formation.

Flax seed oil is an acceptable alternative to salmon oil, but it contains only half the concentration of omega 3 fatty acids. On the other hand, salmon oil contains both families of the omega 3 fats in higher amounts than found in flax seed.

The bottom line is that salmon oil is the "gold standard" as a source of omega 3 fatty acids. In the most difficult cases, a high quality fish oil is essential for shutting chronic inflammation down quickly.

Glutathione

Glutathione supplementation is a good means for combating oxidative stress. Glutathione binds, or conjugates, directly with heavy metals, and in that manner serves as the primary protector of the kidneys. In addition, glutathione functions as an enzymatic antioxidant within a wide variety of cells to prevent or limit secondary damage from free radicals within specialized areas of the cell. In people who are HIV positive, a deficiency of glutathione precedes the onset of AIDS. Thus, glutathione is important not only for detoxification of heavy metals and protection of the inner cell, it is also of vital importance in the control of the most difficult viruses. Glutathione is best absorbed if you open the capsules into water, mix, and drink. The glutathione-water mixture may also be put into an empty nasal spray bottle and sprayed into the nostrils. The glutathione-water mixture stays potent for about 2 hours.

Friendly Bacteria

Did you know that the effective metabolism of food requires that your intestinal lining have a healthy population of friendly bacteria?

We usually think of bacteria as dangerous or unhealthy growths–such as the *Streptococcus* bacteria that gives rise to Strep throat, or rheumatic heart disease. However, there are also friendly bacteria, such as *Lactobacillus acidophilus* or *Bifidobacterium bifidum*–a good population of which is absolutely essential for proper digestion and an infection-free body.

The loss of friendly bacteria is part of the reason why

our country's obsession with antibiotics is so harmful. In fact, the recurring depletion of our needed friendly bacteria may be a significant factor in the increase of many infectious diseases over the past few years. Suspects in this list include *Candida* (yeast), *Salmonella*, and the deadly HUS (hemolytic uremic syndrome) in children which is due to exposure to animal-born *E. coli* infections.

As noted before, within 48 hours after beginning a course of antibiotics, the gut is sterilized. All the healthy bacteria needed to metabolize food are destroyed and a void is created that disease-causing strains of bacteria and yeast find ideal.

This is why we recommend a natural process to eliminate infections rather than antibiotics. Our "Infection-fighting Plan" is available to members of our Health Connection Action Group.

To promote the needed intestinal bacteria, we recommend a good friendly bacteria supplement (which we recommend be taken before breakfast with lemon water, and again during the day with cultured dairy foods). To support the latter, we recommend yogurt, either plain or with the addition of strawberries, red grapes, sunflower seeds and/or pumpkin seeds.

Zinc

Important in bodily repair, zinc is brought into play during the inflammatory response. It helps make SOD and an important antibiotic. Zinc is especially important in men for the production of hormones. Severe zinc deficiency has been shown to cause male sterility. A zinc deficiency may result in smaller sex organs, possibly due to inadequate gonadotropin. Gonadotropin is a hormone, which has a sexually stimulating effect on the sex glands of both the male and female. Sufficient levels of this sex hormone are produced only in the presence of adequate zinc…the production of sperm could not take place without a large amount of zinc.

Zinc depletes rapidly, and when deficient in oral tissue, it is a marker of oxidative stress. Zinc may also decrease a persons susceptibility to colds and infections. Zinc is present in all tissues, organs and secretions of the body. It is essential for cellular reproduction, which is the process of growth and repair. Zinc is found in particularly high concentrations in the prostate and reproductive fluids. It helps prevent the buildup of Vitamin A in the liver. Zinc is also needed to produce liver enzymes.

A man's prostate gland requires significant amounts of zinc (more than can usually be obtained from diet, once depleted). Also, both men and women run short of zinc during chronic inflammation. For this reason zinc is recommended for almost everyone. To be certain, we teach the doctors who provide Free Radical Therapy to do an oral zinc status test. If the result is sufficiently low, a zinc lozenge is recommended in addition to zinc supplementation.

Obtaining Your Supplements

We get calls from people across the country who struggle in their attempts to find quality forms of the required supplements. An example is calcium. Bone meal, oyster shell and dolomite are common ingredients in many calcium supplements, but should all be avoided. While they are legitimate calcium sources, they each have their problems. Bone meal can be a source of lead; oyster shell is nothing more than calcium carbonate (which can cause as many problems as it solves by adding to the free calcium level); and dolomite is simply rock calcium which requires a healthy production of stomach acid. There are better choices.

We most often recommend calcium citrate which is the most alkaline source. However, there is also a potential problem with calcium citrate. You must not take it with any aluminum-based antacids, or you risk adding to the absorption of aluminum. (The answer to this, though, is never to take antacids. For this purpose, turn instead to buttermilk.)

Not all supplements are equal in value, and we constantly evaluate the list of those we recommend. We carry many different brands, and we look first to make sure each is of the right quality for the purposes we outline. Then, we look for the most economical.

Stocking and selling supplements has never been a major objective of ours. However, many of the ones we suggest are difficult to obtain. For this reason, we elected some time ago to begin making select supplements available through our company. We want you to have a place to turn if you are unable to find what you want at your local health food store. In addition, many who seek these supplements either need or desire the convenience of being able to order through us and have the supplements delivered right to their door.

So, if you can't find what you are looking for, if you just don't have time to look, or if you are concerned about getting the right supplements and the best quality, we invite you to place your order with us.

We can have your order to you as fast as the next day. It's your choice. And you won't have to worry about buying the right thing. In addition, we can go to a health food store near us to find any unusual item. For this service, we'll charge a small additional fee over the cost of the item and shipping to you.

Chapter Seven
Required Laboratory Testing

The popular stereotype is that men never ask for directions. Attempting health adjustments without referring to your key blood and urine indices is much like this stereotype–wasted effort without the necessary directions!

Testing falls into two general categories–preliminary testing (normally quick, inexpensive and non-invasive) and formal testing (the key blood and urine indices).

Preliminary Testing

The following are simple and inexpensive tests that can be easily run:

• **To Evaluate pH–The Hydrion pH Test**

The simplest test of all to perform is pH testing using Hydrion pH test strips. Since pH levels reveal the presence of acid stress, the first of the subclinical areas upon which Free Radical Therapy is based, it's especially helpful to be able to do this test simply and quickly. To test your saliva pH, swallow several times beforehand, then touch a piece of the paper to your tongue and wet it with saliva. If you suffer from chemical sensitivities, then you might want to put a small amount of saliva onto a spoon, and touch the test strip to that. Within thirty seconds match the pH strip against the color chart provided with the pH paper. The color correlates with the pH. Since a neutral (7.0) to alkaline (7.5) pH is fundamental to optimum health (and since the test is so easily performed even in your own home), this approach can be readily used. Test strips can be obtained from us, and instructions are included.

- **To Gauge Zinc Levels–The Oral Zinc Status**
  Adequate zinc levels are readily tested through a procedure known as an oral zinc status. A 0.15% solution of zinc sulfate is placed at the rate of one drop every two seconds onto a dry tongue. The solution is initially tasteless. The number of drops before a strong taste occurs is recorded. If taste occurs within the first ten drops, a healthy level of zinc is indicated. Taste occurring within eleven to twenty drops indicates a borderline deficient zinc condition. More than twenty drops indicates an overtly deficient zinc condition.

- **To Evaluate Adequate Levels Of Iodine**
  Apply iodine (2% solution) on clean, dry skin after morning shower. Use skin away from sources of friction from clothing, such as upper thigh or abdomen. Painted area should be about the size of a sliver dollar. Do not use lotion or other skin preparations on this area. Leave stained area of skin alone and check in 12 hours. If the stain is still present after 12 to 24 hours, the body is not deficient in iodine. If the iodine stain has faded or completely absorbed in that time, the body is deficient in iodine. Repeating the above procedure may treat the iodine deficiency. When the iodine is no longer absorbed, the body has obtained enough iodine through the skin and the procedure should be discontinued.

Formal Testing

Our comprehensive health evaluations are based upon the following required blood and urine profiles. Please note that the related dental evaluation and our Free Radical Therapy questionnaire (which includes medical history, diet, lifestyle and supplementation) are also required parts of formal testing.

The Key Blood/Urine Profiles

A laboratory request form is part of our consultations and HealthConnection evaluation. If a voucher for blood work is obtained from our office, your membership in the Action Group is a prerequisite. All of the necessary forms are sent when you arrange to obtain your HealthConnection evaluation or consultation. Once everything is returned to us completely filled out, and once the blood results arrive here, we begin the process of evaluation.

Five "groups" of information are needed then: (1) a blood chemistry analysis, (2) a complete blood count, (3) a urinalysis, (4) a dental evaluation, and (5) the medical history, symptom, diet and lifestyle questionnaire.

The Required Blood Chemistry Analysis

Blood chemistry profiles should include the following serum measurements:

% Saturation (transferrin)

ANA

Albumin

Alkaline Phosphatase

Beta 2 Microglobulin, serum

Beta 2 Microglobulin, urine

Bicarbonate or Carbon Dioxide (HCO_3^- or CO_2)

Bilirubin, total

BUN (Blood Urea Nitrogen)

Calcium

Chloride

Cholesterol

Cortisol

Creatinine

Ferritin

G-6-PD
GGT
Glucose
HDL
Iron
IgA, IgE, IgG, IgM
LDL Cholesterol
LDH
Phosphorous
Potassium
SGOT (AST)
SGPT (ALT)
Sodium
Thyroxine (T4)
TIBC (Total iron binding capacity)
Total Protein
Triglyceride
TSH
Uric Acid

A Simple Way To Order Your Blood Analysis

We've made arrangements with all of the largest clinical laboratories so you can obtain the needed chemistry tests at a significant discount. Contact our office for details. This is available only if you're not planning to use insurance.

If you want to use your insurance, then you must work through your doctor and have the results forwarded to our office. If this is your choice, we would be glad to send you or your doctor a list of the required blood tests.

The Complete Blood Count (CBC)

In addition, a CBC (Complete Blood Count) with a manual differential should also be ordered. These readings give key information regarding the makeup and distribution of your blood cells.

Urinalysis With Microscopic Examination

Finally, a urinalysis should be performed including pH, color, specific gravity, and microscopic examination. This helps us to assess the passage of white and red blood cells, plus bacteria and various sediments, especially crystals.

The Dental Evaluation

We provide a dental evaluation form which prompts your doctor to provide the data we need. We are looking for what we term "A Mouthful of Evidence" of the six fundamental defects in chronic disease. We want to also know the condition of the teeth, the kinds of restorations and appliances, such as amalgam and bridges, as well as the condition of the tongue, lips, muscles of mastication, and gum and mouth tissues, and whether or not you have root canals.

The Medical History, Symptom, Diet, And Lifestyle Questionnaire

This comprehensive questionnaire gives a window into what's going on with you, and provides us with a means of looking for clues into the cause of your problems. Allow at least an hour to complete the questionnaire. The more we know about you and your background, the better we'll be able to get at the cause and develop a strategy for leading you out of the darkened maze of poor health.

A Summary Of What We Need

1. A *blood chemistry analysis* which includes the specific tests listed on this page.

2. A *complete blood count* (CBC) with a manual differential.
3. A *urinalysis* with microscopic examination.
4. A *dental evaluation* per our dental questionnaire.
5. A *lifestyle, diet, and medical history survey* as reported on our comprehensive questionnaire.

Action Group Membership Is Required

Remember, to obtain our consultation services, you must first join our Health Connection Action Group.

Chapter Eight: The Problem With Amalgam
Mercury Poisoning vs. Chronic Mercury Toxicity

The classic medical diagnosis of "mercury poisoning" includes an evaluation of the urine and/or blood mercury level of an unchallenged specimen. A high reading is associated with massive overdose exposure to mercury in its various forms. The result is often of a critical nature, such as inability to breathe, blood pressure and pH instability, or an extreme impairment to the central nervous system.

Minamata Disease
Individuals who suffer from such exposure manifest severe tremors and probably experience convulsions and dementia as well as dysfunction of any or all of the body's major systems. The classic example of this is the Minamata Bay incident in Japan in which an entire village was exposed from eating fish contaminated by a manufacturing plant's mercury waste.

Minamata Disease has since become the official label assigned to people who are poisoned by methyl mercury. The traditional term, *mercury poisoning*, is still used for Minamata Disease, but is also used to describe the effects of acute poisoning from other mercury sources.

Methylmercury, Mercury Vapor And Inorganic Mercury
The American Dental Association conveniently claims that "silver" amalgam fillings do not cause disease because the classic signs of mercury poisoning have

never been demonstrated. This claim is quite accurate, but also misleading. Amalgam fillings do not cause you to be exposed to methylmercury. Rather, amalgam brings about a chronic exposure to two entirely different forms of mercury—mercury vapor and inorganic mercury. (Inorganic mercury exits the fillings and enters the surrounding soft tissues through a process known as oral galvanism, which occurs when the mouth is very acidic. The presence of a purple "tattoo" on the gumline near the filling is evidence of this happening.) The combined effect is much different than what is generally attributed to so-called mercury poisoning. This is true even in the acute poisoning effect of these two mercury species.

Micromercurialism

Poisoning from mercury vapors, termed *micromercurialism,* was described in 1969 by a Russian scientist, I.M. Trachtenburg. (To learn more about the symptoms of micromercurialism, see Appendix Three.) Not surprisingly, micromercurialism, like Minamata Disease, does not accurately describe the effect of chronic, low-dose exposure to the two forms of mercury that arise from amalgam fillings. Making matters worse, people who are exposed to the mercury from dental fillings frequently also receive chronic exposure from other sources. These include methylmercury from fish and a variety of medications such as hemorrhoid preparations. When observed from this light, the symptoms of low-dose, chronic exposure to mercury from a variety of mercury species do not fit any of the patterns of mercury poisoning.

Chronic Mercury Toxicity

To more accurately describe the many overlapping

symptoms of chronic mercury exposure from the various mercury sources, H.L. "Sam" Queen coined the term *chronic mercury toxicity*. This term more accurately describes what is observed in most free living individuals who are exposed not only to the two sources of mercury from dental fillings, but also methyl and phenyl mercury from a variety of other sources.

Chronic mercury toxicity can manifest in a variety of symptoms, but will particularly show up as one or more of the six fundamental, subclinical defects common to all chronic diseases. Through bringing about these subclinical conditions, exposure to mercury from dental fillings may heighten susceptibility to infections and contribute to a host of degenerative diseases, including autoimmune disorders.

**The Truth Regarding The ADA's Claims
Of Amalgam Safety**

The claim by the ADA that mercury from dental fillings must be safe because it does not bring about any of the classic blood, urine, and physical signs of mercury poisoning, intentionally misleads. To the contrary, the combined effect of chronic, low-dose exposure to mercury from amalgam and other sources has the ability to bring about a variety of changes in blood chemistry in the absence of classic signs of poisoning. Those who would like you to believe that mercury is harmful only when it brings about the classic description of mercury poisoning are doing a great disservice to the entire general public.

Chronic mercury toxicity, by bringing about all six of the subclinical defects described earlier in this booklet, looks and acts much different than classic mercury poisoning. One common characteristic is what is often referred to as *mercury retention*. When mercury retention is evident, your urine mercury level reads very near to zero, and the blood level of mercury is low to low normal–even though chronic inflammation may be very strong. (Refer to Appendix Four for a comparison of urine readings.)

Mercury Retention And Free Radical Therapy

The realization that mercury retention is far more common than at first imagined, and the response to this condition with the protocol described by Free Radical Therapy, has helped many people regain their health who otherwise might still be hopelessly lost in the disease maze.

This is even more significant when you realize the combined impact of exposure not only to mercury but to all heavy metals, plus exposure to other hazardous substances. The list includes arsenic from pesticides, lead from paints, and cadmium from acrylics and soldering materials. Free Radical Therapy recognizes this, and provides the key for successfully dealing with these exposures and the health problems that they bring about.

One important advantage of the six subclinical defects/Free Radical Therapy approach to detoxification (and to declining health regardless of the cause), is that it provides a way of dealing with the person who has multiple symptoms. In the past, for instance, when a person had 10 or more symptoms a doctor was left somewhat helpless regarding how to treat him. A doctor's quandary was understandable since the disease model approach demands that only the symptoms be addressed. On the other hand, by categorizing all the symptoms from a Free Radical Therapy perspective–often a must with people who've been chronically exposed to mercury over many years–your doctor gains the only logical means of ever leading them out of the disease maze.

How Serious Is The Exposure From Amalgam?

What most people do not know is that an average mouthful of amalgams–about 8 mercury-silver restorations–can generate mercury vapor readings greater than 50 micrograms per cubic meter of air. Is this a lot? The Threshold Limit Value (TLV) as established by various government agencies throughout the world, including the U.S.A., is 50 micrograms per cubic meter of air. (To see how the amount of exposure to the mercury vapors of amalgam fillings compares with other sources of exposure, and with the various world government limits, see Appendix Four.)

There are other exposure avenues in addition to mercury vapor in the air we breathe. For instance, mercury can be absorbed through the skin, which generally happens only if you handle it (which you should never do). Exposure also results from swallowing mercury (a danger when amalgam is being placed in your teeth).

Swallowed mercury may or may not get absorbed. It nevertheless has the potential of compromising your health by first killing the friendly bacteria in your intestines that keep you free from infections, and which otherwise help digest a variety of foods. Mercury has also been shown to encourage the growth of bacteria that are (or can become) resistant to antibiotics.

Among mercury exposure sources, however, mercury vapor is the most common. Further, mercury vapor from amalgam is *the* major exposure for most individuals.

It is interesting that no level of mercury exposure, vapor or otherwise, has ever been shown to be safe. In addition, it's important to keep in mind that the Threshold Limit Value is OSHA's arbitrary level for "hitting the panic button." Sweden has established lower levels (25 micrograms per cubic meter of air) as the point it considers dangerous.

For most people the anxiety-generating aspect of all this is the insidious nature of mercury exposure from amalgam fillings: It's in your mouth and it's with you all the time.

Incontrovertible Points Regarding Amalgam

People always ask, "Am I being exposed to mercury from my dental fillings? Am I being exposed enough to compromise my health? Should I have them taken out?" To answer this let's refer to a few points which can no longer be disputed:

* Mercury is a poison.
* Dental amalgam fillings are comprised of approximately 50% mercury.
* Mercury leaks from dental amalgam over the lifetime of a filling.
* The leakage is most pronounced when you eat, chew food, drink hot liquids, or when you grind your teeth at night.
* Mercury continues to leak for up to 90 minutes following disruption of the amalgam surface by chewing.
* Mercury from dental fillings has been traced to every organ and tissue in the body, and most definitely crosses the placental barrier in pregnant females.
* There is no level of mercury that scientists have ever declared to be safe.
* Mercury from fillings has been shown to bring about kidney dysfunction.
* Mercury from fillings has been shown to encourage the growth of antibiotic resistant bacteria.

Gaining A Basis For An Informed Decision

The American Dental Association (ADA) appears to be doing everything it can to keep you from knowing about these incontrovertible points. On the other hand, Health Canada, the national health insurance provider for all Canadians, recognizes these points and has now placed limits on amalgam for the people of Canada.

An informed decision regarding whether to keep your amalgams requires that you not limit your investigation to the advice of a trade organization (the ADA) that has everything to lose if its members are forced to find an alternative material. It's important that you look elsewhere, which is why we've included this chapter.

Those wishing to get a very detailed, technical presentation on mercury toxicity can order Sam Queen's *Chronic Mercury Toxicity: New Hope Against An Endemic Disease,* which was the first medical reference book ever written on this topic.

Dealing With Hazardous Exposure Related Health Problems

Individuals concerned about dealing more specifically with health problems due to exposure to mercury and/or other hazardous materials may wish to make an appointment with one of the doctors who have attended Sam Queen's seminars, or draw upon our *IV-C Mercury Tox Program* publication (*A Guide For The Patient*). Or, if you desire health guidance that is tailored to your particular situation, our consultation services through either the verbal Consultation or the written HealthConnection personal health evaluation are suggested options.

Determining Individual Exposure Levels

Due to the pressure exerted by those who wish to

hide or downplay the issue, the American public still is generally unaware that commonly used amalgam dental fillings expose people to mercury.

In order to overcome this, concerned health care practitioners have resorted to a number of means to demonstrate individual exposure levels.

The Jerome Mercury Vapor Analyzer

We believe the clearest presentation of mercury exposure from amalgam on an individual basis is through the correct use of the mercury vapor analyzer. In our experience, the most reliable piece of equipment of this type is the Jerome Mercury Vapor Analyzer.

Unfortunately, confusion has arisen regarding this instrument. The readings demonstrate only mercury vapor exposure (a hazard), not mercury toxicity (a clinical condition).

Mercury vapor analyzers were originally developed for geological surveys where the user was prospecting for gold. Gold has a strong affinity for mercury. Thus, wherever there is gold ore, mercury vapor is close by. Later, because of the instrument's high sensitivity, OSHA began using the mercury vapor analyzer to evaluate hazards in the workplace. It is capable of determining the amount of mercury vapor in micrograms (millionths of a gram) per cubic meter of air.

The Significance Of Very Small Quantities Of Mercury

Since there are approximately 28.5 grams in an ounce, a millionth of a gram doesn't seem like much. It is important to understand, however, how incredibly toxic and dangerous mercury vapor actually is (even in extremely small quantities). This is why OSHA routinely uses the machine to evaluate the environment in which workers must spend their day.

Keep in mind that 50 micrograms per cubic meter of air has been established as the U.S. Government's limit for the workplace. What this means is that any environment which exceeds this level of exposure over an 8-hour workday is considered unsafe and–if humans were required to work in that space–should be shut down.

What is shocking for most people to realize is that it is simple–through the use of a mercury vapor analyzer–to demonstrate that the oral environment of individuals who have amalgam fillings frequently approaches or exceeds the government's workplace limit.

When such measurement is performed to gather research information, and when the person being tested is fully informed by the practitioner of the functional and ethical limitations imposed by this procedure, then mercury vapor analysis is appropriate.

Mercury Exposure vs. Mercury Toxicity

Again, however, a careful distinction needs to be made here: Exposure to mercury vapor (a hazard) does not equal mercury toxicity (a medical condition). The fact of exposure alone does not mean a person has mercury toxicity.

On the other hand, the fact of exposure does clearly present that there is a hazard. And the hazard, of course, is that no level of mercury is safe. Based on this, any exposure to mercury that is continual, or repeated over several months, could eventually lead to a medical condition, depending on the tissues or organs most directly affected.

In fairness to those who have argued on the side of the ADA, and against the dangers of mercury exposure from amalgam, we want to emphasize that the public should not be led to a premature medical conclusion.

Conversely, the ADA should not allow its trade members to place amalgam without informing patients of the same incontrovertible points we have made in this book against mercury.

At the very least, exposure to mercury vapor should be clearly explained and presented as an undesirable and hazardous event. In all cases (in agreement with the World Health Organization), exposure to mercury should be minimized and–if possible–eliminated.

Why The Debate?

When the exposure is so clearly demonstrated–and when the hazard from exposure is so great–why is there any debate at all?

Frankly, the answer is that there is a lot at stake. Dental tradesmen who place amalgam, and who may not have the skill to place the more technique-sensitive restorative materials, could be out of work. The ADA holds a patent on amalgam, and thereby has a financial stake in the debate. Further, a great number of people in prestigious and affluent positions could lose their status if they admit that amalgam, as a dental restorative material in the patient's mouth, is hazardous.

The ADA's History

Few people realize that the ADA was formed in the mid-1800's specifically for the purpose of supporting the position of dentists who wished to use amalgam as a dental restorative material.

Amalgam was introduced in America from France during the 1830's. The existing Dental Association, which was run primarily by medical doctors, denounced the material as unsafe and pressured those who practiced dentistry not to use it. Alternative materials, however, were expensive, more difficult to use and/or ineffective as dental restoratives.

The demands of economics and ease of use won out. The predecessor dental association collapsed, and the American Dental Association was born with an agenda specifically supporting the promotion and use of amalgam in dentistry.

Several times since the 1830's, concerned dentists have vigorously opposed the continued use of amalgam. In each case, the ADA has utilized its growing political and economic clout to squelch the objections and the objectors.

The ADA Is A Trade Organization, Not A Research Institute!

Let's take a closer look at the American Dental Association and its function as an organization. To begin with, the ADA is a trade organization and not a research institute. Its major function is to *promote the image and effectiveness* of its member dentists *and their practices* to the American public.

ADA Similarities To Other Trade Organizations

The ADA's actions regarding mercury exposure from amalgam are consistent with other trade organizations. Again, trade organizations tend to promote specific commercial causes which benefit their memberships. Carried to an extreme, this would seem to indicate that image is more important than public safety.

In this regard, the ADA holds some similarity to the International Tobacco Growers' Association. The American Tobacco Growers' Association is also a trade organization. Of course, its primary function is the promotion of tobacco use. Considering the overwhelming evidence demonstrating harm from smoking, most of us cringe at the idea of an organization promoting this habit.

However, it's important to keep in mind that smoking as a hazard has only become a widely-held view by the American public during recent years. It took a lot of effort to overcome the tobacco lobby's powerful economics, politics, and advertising.

Prior to this time, smoking was seen as a social event and was touted for its "calming" effects. It should also be noted that, even though most people understand that tobacco use is a health risk, the tobacco industry continues—even now—to insist that smoking is safe (although, under pressure, they admit that it is addicting). In much the same way the ADA continues to insist that amalgam use is safe.

The ADA's "Efforts" To Inform People That Amalgam Contains Mercury

In the recent past there have been those who thought that the ADA would respond to the growing body of science suggesting that amalgam is not safe by (at least) informing the American public that there is mercury in amalgam.

The ADA's "efforts" to "inform" the American public that mercury is a major ingredient in amalgam is primarily limited to providing information on their web site, which we've reprinted in Appendix One. The information strongly downplays the inherent danger presented by the mercury contained in amalgam.

Rather than inform the American public that amalgam contains mercury, the ADA has brought tremendous pressure on its member doctors to keep them from fully discussing mercury in amalgam with their patients. More than this, the ADA has attempted to make it "illegal" or "unethical" for a dentist to elect to practice mercury (or amalgam) free.

A widespread proclamation to the American public

that mercury is in amalgam would be a start, of course, but much more is needed. The ADA needs to make a pronouncement that–as the research clearly demonstrates–mercury not only escapes from amalgam but also causes a needless exposure to an enormously hazardous material.

Neither of these pronouncements is likely to ever be made by the ADA. Instead, they are busy trying to develop replacement restorative materials, such as high copper amalgam, hoping that mercury amalgam will just be phased out and forgotten. That's why it's important that you learn of these facts, and why helping people deal with potential mercury problems is an important part of what we do.

Why Nothing Has Been Done

Here are some possible reasons for inaction:

First, if amalgam were banned today it has been estimated that 30-35% of the dentists would not have the skills necessary to continue practicing (using alternative materials). This is because amalgam is the easiest material to place in a tooth requiring basic restoration. Logically, dentists who build their practice on amalgam may do so because they lack the skills to move on to the better materials. It would appear that, as members of a trade organization, these dentists depend on the ADA's power to keep them in business.

Second, if amalgam were banned today by the government (we say government, because the ADA is unlikely to "sound the alarm"), then lawyers would immediately begin swarming all over the issue. The lawsuits and redistribution of wealth and power which could result would be monumental.

A health panic could ensue, the courts would likely become clogged with litigation, and some major manufacturers and insurance companies would probably be ruined. The potential economic impact should not be taken lightly. Some of the extended business entities involved in amalgam production, distribution, and delivery are economic heavyweights. The ripple effect from the disruption of these companies–combined with potential wide scale litigation–could result in an economic catastrophe.

Of course, the government could step in proactively and set up a framework of protection to overcome or minimize the damage to business in America as usual.

In order to establish a moratorium, however, elected and appointed officials would have to step beyond the reach of some of our nation's most powerful political lobbies: the dental and medical professions, the major manufacturers and, ultimately, the insurance companies which back them all.

The Likely Result...

Given the economic and political environment in which our society functions, it is exceedingly unlikely that any of the above will ever take place.

Instead the following scenario is more likely. The dental profession will gradually replace its reliance upon amalgam with non-mercury based materials. This has already begun. Over the last ten years the ADA has sanctioned a number of composites (dental fillings which do not contain mercury) for a wide range of uses as restorative materials. Included in this list is a new non-mercury amalgam, composed of gallium, indium, and tin, which has (in November 1996) been granted the ADA Seal of Acceptance by the Council on Scientific Affairs. Known as *Galloy*, the product is as easy to place as mercury amalgam. This helps to guarantee that the tradesmen will have something to work with should their worst case scenario (the banning of amalgam) become a reality for them.

But who will come to the rescue of those already harmed by amalgam? No one. The people will be left without any recourse. Then, if the ADA's plan goes as it would probably prefer, in seventy-five years or so, the mercury issue will probably just go away.

Who Will Pay The Price?

As it stands now, those wishing to replace existing amalgam restorations do so out of their own pockets. Since the ADA does not recognize mercury from amalgam as a hazard, replacing amalgams with composites is only an "elective cosmetic option." Per the ADA, your dentist cannot ethically replace amalgam unless you either document that the reason is for appearance alone (composites <u>do</u> look more like your natural teeth), or you produce a diagnosis from a medical doctor requiring amalgam removal. Of course, no insurance company covers discretionary cosmetic dentistry.

Further, by having the amalgam replaced for cosmetic purposes, you implicitly agree that no harm has come from the amalgam. Under this scenario, all the major players–the dental and medical professions, the manufacturers, the insurance companies, and the politicians and government officials who have gone along with this approach–completely escape any responsibility for the hazard created by mercury from amalgam.

Those exposed will deal with the health results on their own (unless they can get an extremely hard-to-come-by medical diagnosis of mercury toxicity).

It's a functional solution, unless of course, it's you or someone you care about who is being affected!

For More Information on Mercury

In addition to reading the Institute for Health Realities publications, you can learn more about mercury at the following web sites:

http://www.testfoundation.org

http//www.bodyburden.org

Chapter Nine: Health Consultations
with the Institute for Health Realities

Tell Me About Individualized Health Evaluations

One prerequisite is necessary in order to obtain an individualized health evaluation through our company: membership in the HealthConnection Action Group. In some states, a local doctor's signature may be needed to get blood work done.

Action Group Membership

Membership in the HealthConnection Action Group is the necessary first step in order to obtain consultations and health evaluations. In addition to gaining access to consultations, members receive a number of other important benefits and discounts. All of these efforts help Action Group Members remain on the cutting edge of the Free Radical Therapy information highway.

There is a powerful rationale behind Action Group membership, and we want you to understand it. Concentrating our consultation efforts on those who are better informed is essential in light of our diminishing time resources. Frankly, time demands make it necessary that our consulting team limit its work to those who understand Health Model concepts. In addition, those who participate in the Action Group, actively support Free Radical Therapy research.

Joining the Action Group provides members with the following benefits:

- A complimentary copy of *Your Personal Health Guide*.
- The option of receiving our free electronic magazine. These e-zine is like a mini seminar with Sam Queen. Past topics have included coral calcium,

detox essentials, free iron, and an immune-building strategy.

- Exclusive access to professional health consultations. As noted before, Action Group membership is required in order to obtain consultations. Once membership is obtained, the initial HealthConnection or Consultation evaluations are available at their usual fee. Action Group membership is also required for those who have already obtained HealthConnection or Consultation evaluations and who are now seeking follow-up consultations.

- Advance information on upcoming research, publications and course offerings. You'll know about our research, seminars, publications and computer software developments before anyone else.

- Savings on food supplement purchases. Action Group members receive a discount on food supplement purchases.

- Participation in the Action Group health movement. Our research and health efforts are furthered by Action Group members. Availability of supplements to the public, access to mercury-free dentistry, and the promotion of *Health Realities*-related research all are supported by our Action Group members.

A Doctor's Prescription

In addition to required Action Group membership, in some states, blood work is only available with your doctor's signature or prescription. Forms and information from our office will help your doctor understand our program, and can aid you in obtaining your prescription.

If you don't have a local doctor, call our office and we'll see if we know of a good practitioner in your area.

Now that the requirements to obtain personalized

health evaluations are out of the way, let's describe the consultations themselves:

All levels include:
• An evaluation of your health/dental questionnaire and chemistries
• A written action plan of health and lifestyle recommendations
• A one-year subscription to the HealthConnection Action Group (HCAG)

Level 1 – General Health Assessment

We recommend this level if you have no known health problems, feel relatively healthy and have not had any serious disease or illness. This level includes the key blood chemistries that insurance companies would review to evaluate for a life insurance plan. This is the place to start if you want to begin plans to maintain your health throughout your life.

Your package will include:
• A basic blood chemistry voucher to take to your local laboratory
• A half-hour of audio-taped information, background and suggestions

Level 2 – Full Consultation

This level provides a comprehensive chemistry-based approach to improving nearly all health conditions except cancer. (If cancer concerns you, either because you want to prevent it, or have already been diagnosed, you will want to begin with Level 3.) If you already have a known disease condition, are taking multiple prescription drugs, have high blood pressure, suffer from repeat infections or a combination of symptoms (for example, heart disease and periodontal disease) we suggest you begin at this level. This extensive blood chemistry, customized for the Institute, allows for an overall approach to your health.

An oral evaluation and report is based upon the required blood and urine tests, plus the information gained from our intensive questionnaire. Once we've gone over the data, a phone consultation is arranged, or if you prefer, you may have the consultation in our office. An audiotape of the consultation and an Action Plan is provided to assist you in your review of the consultation.

A Full Consultation allows you to pursue a tailored approach to detoxification or health improvement, and provides your health care professional additional and valuable insight into your condition.

Your package will include:

• A comprehensive blood chemistry voucher to take to your local laboratory

• A one-hour initial phone or on-site consultation with Sam

• An audio-taped report

• Discounts on further follow-up chemistries and consultations

Level 3 – Immune Building Program

If you have been diagnosed with cancer, are at high risk for cancer (such as with family history, exposure to toxins, etc.), or are concerned about cancer risk for any reason, this is the level for you. It includes all of Level 2 as well as specific chemistries designed to understand the basis of cancer and how best to combat it. This level utilizes the maximum effort to rebuild your immune system, and is ideal for people who have already undergone chemotherapy, radiation or surgery, since this level is excellent for monitoring your progress.

Your package will include:
- A blood chemistry voucher to take to your local laboratory for the tests
- A one-and-one-half-hour phone or on-site consultation with Sam
- An audio-taped report
- Discounts on follow-up chemistries and consultations

Level 4 – HealthConnection™

This comprehensive written health evaluation and subsequent action plan is the "Cadillac" of our consultation services. Although based upon the same extensive criteria as the Full Consultation, you receive in addition a full written report that evaluates the data, relating it to the six fundamental defects. It also evaluates the data relative to footprints of toxic exposure, risk for infection, anemia, cancer, heart disease, immune status, chronic or active inflammation, kidney and adrenal function, liver and bone status, mercury toxicity, and the risk for a host of degenerative diseases.

The HealthConnection report is truly individualized. Your written, personal evaluation includes an Action Program uniquely tailored to your health needs. You're clearly told exactly what to do, what to take, and when.

The evaluation is particularly useful for archiving your health status at a current point in time. This allows you to apprise multiple doctors of your health status so that everyone you work with is thinking along the same lines. In addition, the HealthConnection includes a 30-minute consultation to make sure everything is clear to you or your doctor.

Your package will include:
- A comprehensive blood chemistry voucher to take to your local laboratory

• A half-hour audio-taped report
• A 30-minute phone or on-site consultation with Sam to help clear up details, which is also audio-taped
• An archived comprehensive health report detailing current health as well as probable risk for future illness
• Discounts on further follow-up chemistries and consultations

Conclusion

An ancient proverb says that even the longest journey begins with but a single step. Of equal importance, that first step must be in the right direction, or you'll never reach your intended goal. *Your Personal Health Guide* is meant to make certain you reach the health goal you're seeking. Thus, this book is not only an important first step, but a conceptually correct first step that empowers you to help yourself and those you love enough to invite along on the trip.

We want to encourage you regarding your journey. Gaining and retaining good health is obviously a life-long pursuit, but it doesn't have to be unpleasant. There is great joy in attaining a fuller life and in sharing this gift with others.

Each of us has an inner circle, an inside group of those for whom we care deeply. If you value these special people, then you'll give them the best "you" that you can be...and you'll help them to achieve the same goal.

We all could use a personal guide in this quest. As you find and apply the truth about health and life, then you become a living guide for others. In this way you transform yourself into so much more than a printed page could ever be. Through this process you express the ultimate purpose of *Your Personal Health Guide*.

Appendix One
ADA Amalgam Position Paper

The following information is the American Dental Association's position on amalgam. It is included to give you the opportunity to more readily evaluate both sides of the amalgam toxicity issue. The views of the ADA as presented below are <u>not</u> those of the Institute for Health Realities.

ADA Statement on Dental Amalgam

Revised January 8, 2002

Dental amalgam (silver filling) is considered a safe, affordable and durable material that has been used to restore the teeth of more than 100 million Americans. It contains a mixture of metals such as silver, copper and tin, in addition to mercury, which chemically binds these components into a hard, stable and safe substance. Dental amalgam has been studied and reviewed extensively, and has established a record of safety and effectiveness.

Issued in late 1997, the FDI World Dental Federation and the World Health Organization consensus statement on dental amalgam stated, "No controlled studies have been published demonstrating systemic adverse effects from amalgam restorations." The document also states that, aside from rare instances of local side effects of allergic reactions, "the small amount of mercury released from amalgam restorations, especially during placement and removal, has not been shown to cause any ... adverse health effects."

The ADA's Council on Scientific Affairs' 1998 report on its review of the recent scientific literature on amalgam states: "The Council concludes that, based on available scientific information, amalgam continues to be a safe and effective restorative material." The Council's report also states, "There currently appears to be no justification for discontinuing the use of dental amalgam."

In an article published in the February 1999 issue of the Journal of the American Dental Association, researchers report finding "no significant association of Alzheimer's Disease with the number, surface area or history of having dental amalgam restorations" and "no statistically significant differences in brain mercury levels between subjects with Alzheimer's Disease and control subjects."

The U.S. Public Health Service issued a report in 1993 stating there is no health reason not to use amalgam, except in the extremely rare case of the patient who is allergic to a component of amalgam. This supports the findings of the Food and Drug Administration (FDA), the National Institutes of Health Technology Assessment Conference and the National Institute of Dental and Craniofacial Research, that dental amalgam is a safe and effective restorative material. In addition, in 1991, Consumer Reports noted, "Given their solid track record . . . amalgam fillings are still your best bet."

In 1991, the FDA's Dental Products Panel found no valid data to demonstrate clinical harm to patients from amalgams or that having them removed would prevent adverse health effects or reverse the course of existing diseases. The FDA's most recent reaffirmation of amalgam's safety was published on December 31, 2002.

The reaffirmation reads, "FDA and other organizations of the U.S. Public Health Service (USPHS) continue to investigate the safety of amalgams used in dental restorations (fillings). However, no valid scientific evidence has ever shown that amalgams cause harm to patients."

It continues, "Also, USPHS scientists analyzed about 175 peer-reviewed studies submitted in support of three citizen petitions received by FDA after the 1993 report. They concluded that data in these studies did not support claims that individuals with dental amalgam restorations will experience problems, including neurologic, renal or developmental effects, except for rare allergic or hypersensitivity reactions."

The U.S. Public Health Service found in 1993 "no persuasive reason to believe that avoiding amalgams or having them removed will have a beneficial effect on health." In fact, it is inadvisable to have amalgams removed unnecessarily because it can cause structural damage to healthy teeth.

The ADA supports ongoing research in the development of new materials that it hopes will someday prove to be as safe and effective as dental amalgam. However, the ADA continues to believe that amalgam is a valuable, viable and safe choice for dental patients and concurs with the findings of the U.S. Public Health Service that amalgam has "continuing value in maintaining oral health."

Page Updated: January 08, 2003

Those wishing to correspond with the ADA regarding this information may do so at the following address:

American Dental Association
211 East Chicago Avenue
Chicago, IL 60611
www.ada.org

Appendix Two
Making Whole Grain Cereal
And The Egg Cocktail

We recommend the increase of early morning protein through the intake of eggs and whole grains. Eggs constitute the standard for protein quality. Two eggs for breakfast are ideal for weight control, detoxification and overall health. Egg cholesterol is generally no problem as long as you are taking vitamin C, getting good bowel action every day (two or more daily movements that are soft to semisoft), and eating a high fiber diet from whole grains, lentils, fruits, and vegetables. Eggs can be alternately cooked one day and eaten raw the next, providing you are eating cultured dairy every day and taking a supplement of friendly bacteria. If you meet these qualifications, the raw egg cocktail can be prepared as follows:

The Egg Cocktail
Place 4 ounces of unfiltered apple juice in a blender. Add 2 raw eggs, 1 tablespoon plain (unsweetened) yogurt, 1 tablespoon raw sunflower seeds, 1 tablespoon liquid lecithin, 1 tablespoon brewer's yeast flakes, and 1-2 drops of vanilla flavoring or stevia. Blend well. Drink, or pour over the whole grain cereal.

Whole Grain Cereal
To control cholesterol and obtain adequate fiber along with natural Vitamin E for detoxification, make the following breakfast cereal:

Wash, and place in a large cooking pot: 2 cups short grain sweet brown rice, 1 cup millet, 1/2 cup barley, and 1 cup whole grain rye. (If you are sensitive to gluten, you can omit the rye and barley.) Cover with water to 1/2 inch above the grains. Cook at low heat until the grains have absorbed all the water–stirring often to prevent sticking or burning. A little extra water may be needed before the grains are cooked through–a taste test will suffice here. When done, the cooked grains can be stored in the refrigerator. Some should be eaten each day. The cereal can be eaten hot or cold; and fruit, honey, and/or cinnamon can be added. The egg cocktail can be poured over the cereal. On days eggs are cooked, the grains can be eaten by simply adding raw apple juice and heating the mixture; this gives the cereal a pleasantly sweet taste. Unsweetened rice or soy milk or acidophilus low-fat milk can be used. A teaspoon of plain, unsweetened yogurt added to the milk can make it even more effective.

Cooking Whole Grain Cereals

Since these cereals tend to stick to the bottom of your pan and burn, cook them at a very low heat over a longer period of time. Our approach is to bring water to a boil (about twice as much water as the uncooked cereal) and then remove the pan from the heat. Turn the burner to its lowest setting, stir in the cereal, cover the pan, and place it back on the heat. Stir it often for the first few minutes, and let it cook until done and the cereal is no longer watery. Then stir it, remove it from the heat and let it stand for about five minutes.

Appendix Three
Micromercurialism vs.
Chronic Mercury Toxicity

Micromercurialism–a term coined by Trachtenberg[1] to describe the effect of chronic exposure to mercury vapor.
Common symptoms:
- asthenic-vegetative syndrome of unspecific symptoms and signs
- generalized weakness
- fatigue
- anorexia
- weight loss
- gastrointestinal disturbances
- erethism (shyness, loss of memory, personality changes, hyperexcitability, insomnia, and depression)

Some of the more severe symptoms:
- characteristic mercurial tremor
  fine muscular tremor (fingers, lips, eyelids)
  coarse shaking movements
- delirium
- hallucination
- gingivitis
- ptyalism
- ALS-like symptoms[2]

---

[1] Trachtenberg, I.M., "The Chronic Action Of Mercury On The Organism, Current Aspects Of The Problem On Micromercurialism And Its Prophylaxis," *Zdorv'ja Kiev* (Russian) 21: 7-10, 1969.

[2] Vroom, F.Q., and Greer, M., "Mercury Vapor Intoxication," *Brain* 95: 305-18, 1972.

Chronic Mercury Toxicity–a term coined by H.L. "Sam" Queen[3] to describe the combined effect of chronic exposure to mercury from all sources, but especially from dental fillings. Dental amalgam, which constitutes the greatest source of human exposure to mercury, causes the wearer to be exposed to mercury vapor (Hg0) as well as elemental oxidized mercuric ion (Hg2+), with the possibility of exposure to methylmercury from the action of cyanocobalamin on the mercuric ion.

---

[3] Queen, H.L., *Chronic Mercury Toxicity: New Hope Against an Endemic Disease*, Queen and Company, Colorado Springs, CO, 80949-9308, 1988.

Appendix Four
Mercury Vapor Exposure
Sources, Limits, and Thresholds

Average Daily Human Mercury Intake Per Source[1,2]

dental amalgam fillings (mercury vapor)[3]	3.0-17.5 mcg/day
average	10 mcg/day
extremes	100 mcg/day
ADA's calculation[4]	1.0-2.0 mcg/day[5]
fish (methylmercury)	2.4 mcg/day
nonfish food (inorganic mercury)	0.3 mcg/day
air, water, and food	3.09 mcg/day
other sources	negligible

U.S.E.P.A. National Emission Standard for Hazardous
 Air Pollutants 1 mcg/m^3
U.S.E.P.A. Intake Standard for public health,
 not to exceed 20 mcg/day
U.S. NAVY Submarine Limits 10 mcg/m^3
N.I.O.S.H. Govt. Standard[6] 50 mcg/m^3
 (not to be exceeded)
OSHA Threshold Limit Value 50 mcg/m^3
 (indoor air limit for the workplace
 per 8-hour work week)

Max Allowable Concentration 50 mcg/m^3
The Reinhardt relationship between air concentration
exposure and earliest symptoms[7]
abnormal reflexes 10 mcg/m^3
weight loss, appetite loss, shyness 50 mcg/m^3

Harris and Hohenemser's mercury vapor exposure/
clinical symptom relationships[8]

appetite loss, insomnia	10-27 mcg/m^3
hyperthyroidism	10-50 mcg/m^3
abnormal reflexes	100 mcg/m^3
chronic neural disorder	800 mcg/m^3

---

[1] W.H.O. report by Lars Friberg, D.D.S., and Thomas W. Clarkson, Ph.D., M.D. (Hon.), in a preliminary report of their findings before the FDA Panel on Dental Affairs, Convened March 15, 1991 in Rockville, MD.

[2] W.H.O. Report: Environmental Health Criteria 118: Inorganic Mercury, Geneva, 1991.

[3] Vimy, M.J., Lorscheider, F.L., "Dental Amalgam Mercury Daily Dose Estimated From Intra-Oral Vapor Measurements: A Predictor Of Mercury Accumulation In Human Tissues," *J Trace Elem Exp Med* 3: 111-23, 1990.

[4] Arrived at by the ADA using Vimy's data and some very creative math.

[5] Mackert, J.R., Olsson, S., Bergman, S., and Berglund, A., *JADA*, and M. Molin, *Swedish Dental Journal.*

[6] Summary of NIOSH recommendations for occupational health standards. October 1978. Cincinnati, National Institute for Occupational Safety and Health, 1978..

[7] Reinhardt, J.W., "Risk Assessment Of Mercury Exposure From Dental Amalgams," *J Pub Health Dentistry* 28 (3): 1988.

[8] Harris, R.C., and Hohenemser, C., "Mercury: Measuring And Managing The Risk," *Environment* 20(9): 25-36, 1978.

Key Word Index